When Your Doctor has Bad News

In order to protect the privacy rights of my patients, most names in this book and some details surrounding patient stories have been changed. Any real names in patient stories have been used with permission. These real names can be recognized by the use of both first and last names when a patient's story is discussed.

When Your Doctor Has Bad News

Simple Steps *to* Strength, Healing & Hope

Al B. Weir, M.D.

Foreword by
Joni Eareckson Tada

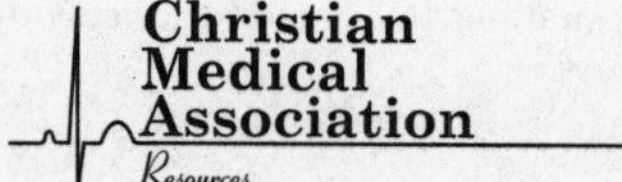

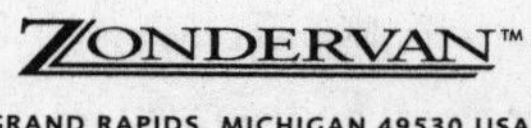

GRAND RAPIDS, MICHIGAN 49530 USA

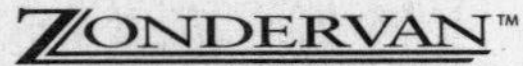

When Your Doctor Has Bad News

Requests for information should be addressed to:
Zondervan, *Grand Rapids, Michigan 49530*

Library of Congress Cataloging-in-Publication Data

Weir, Al. B. (Alva B.), 1951–
When your doctor has bad news : simple steps to strength, healing, and hope / Al. B. Weir III.– 1st ed.
p. cm.
ISBN-10: 0-310-24742-X (softcover)
ISBN-13: 978-0-310-24742-5 (softcover)
1. Sick—Psychology. 2. Medicine—Religious aspects—Christianity.
I. Title.
R726.5.W45 2003
2003003972

Interior design by Todd Sprague
Printed in the United States of America

05 06 07 08 09 10 /❖ DC/ 10 9 8 7 6 5 4

Contents

Before You Begin

I have to admit, the title almost makes me cringe. That's because the doctor once brought me bad news. Very bad news. More than thirty-five years ago, I was lying face up on a hospital bed wondering when the numbness in my body would wear off. I was anxious to get back the use of my hands and legs. I didn't have to wonder long. A tall man in a white coat walked up to my bed, flipped a few pages on his clipboard, looked at me over his glasses, and announced, "Miss Eareckson, your paralysis is permanent."

Like I said, it was bad news. It would have helped a little had the person with the clipboard been Dr. Al Weir—a little empathetic . . . a little less rushed . . . and with a much better sense of timing.

As patients we sometimes look at doctors as though they are the be-all, end-all to our problems, as though they are the secret repositories of all wisdom where it concerns a good or bad medical diagnosis. When my doctor told me that I would never walk again, that I would never be able to hold anyone's hand and feel it, I was devastated. He may as well have blown out the light at the end of my tunnel. After I received the news, I sank into a deep and dark depression. Only years later would I discover the hope and help that has sustained me all these years.

This is what I love about the insights and wisdom of Dr. Weir. In this wonderful new book, we have the chance to sit down with a skilled and respected health-care professional as he opens his heart. Dr. Weir takes the doctor's role a giant step beyond average white-lab-coat responsibilities and guides the reader—especially the one who has received bad news—past the soul-numbing shock of a dismal medical report. He reminds us of the soothing comfort available in the Word of God, of the heart-warming precepts upon which we can build a new life, and of the simple steps a family can take to promote hope and healing.

For too long the health-care industry has been just that—an *industry.* I am grateful to God for doctors like Al Weir who are reestablishing the cherished and time-honored relationship between a doctor and his or her patient. I applaud every effort of people like Dr. Weir who do more—much more—than relate to their patient and the family on a fee-per-service basis. The book you hold in your hand, *When Your Doctor Has Bad News,* not only will help you to navigate the confusing clutter of hospital-related rules and routines but, more than that, will be an invaluable resource for rebuilding the life of your family.

You just may discover that the news you've received from your doctor is not as devastating as you thought, because you just might find God in the midst of it all.

—Joni Eareckson Tada

Winter 2002

ONE

Bad News: Broken Dreams

"Meet me at the emergency room. Hurry, it's Catherine."

Life changes in a heartbeat. As a doctor treating cancer patients, I thought I had learned that tragedy comes to all someday. But I never really brought the lesson home until it was my turn to take the call. In a span of mere seconds, while I was driving my son to football practice, the urgent priorities of my day evaporated.

"Catherine's been hurt, Al. Her back is injured, and she can't get up."

"I'll drop off Bowen and meet you at the emergency room."

While my car raced to the emergency room, my mind raced back to the flame tree that had stretched its lime green arms over most of our backyard in Africa, separating us from the dense jungle beyond it. Soon after our arrival there, I had fashioned a swing with a single rope hung from a great limb of that tree supporting a wooden board for a seat. When Catherine was about one year old, I would gently swing her in that seat beneath the bright red flame tree flowers. She was agile enough to hold the rope, and I was foolishly proud of her agility.

One day I was a bit too aggressive with my push, and I frightened Catherine. She looked back at me as the swing was moving forward and let go of the rope to reach for me with both hands. Immediately, she tipped over backward and went headfirst for the ground. Instead of falling, however, she hooked her ankles around the rope and swung upside down, as safe as a monkey hanging by its tail, until I wrapped my arms around her.

That incredible agility remained with her for the next fourteen years. When we returned to the States, Catherine became a gymnast. Year after year, for hours every day, she progressed through the ranks to reach level ten in competition by the time she was thirteen. When Catherine was fifteen years old, prior to the accident, the biggest decision in her life was whether to home school so she could advance to elite status in gymnastics.

As I raced toward the emergency room, reality gripped my heart. Our lives had just changed. When I arrived, Catherine was lying on her side in great pain.

She told me, "I lost where I was and I bailed out. I knew I was in trouble. When I landed on my shoulders, my legs flexed over my head, and I felt my back snap. I thought, 'Oh my God! I'm going to be paralyzed!'"

The first thing I did was to check her legs. She could move them both. I then ran my hand over her back and found a firm knot over her mid-spine. Walking beside her, I kept my hand on her shoulder as they wheeled her on a stretcher to radiology. The X-ray pictures frightened this doctor daddy, and all I could say was, "Oh my God, please." I contacted the best pediatric spine doctors in Memphis, who happened to be the best pediatric spine doctors in the country. We looked at the MRI together and saw the bone pressing against Catherine's spinal cord at T-11. One more millimeter and my fifteen-year-old daughter would be paralyzed for life.

This was *my* daughter. Just this morning Catherine had been a great gymnast, looking toward a college scholarship and perhaps the Olympics. Now she might be paralyzed for life.

Each of us at some time in our lives will face a doctor or pick up the phone and receive bad news. What do you do when you receive bad

news that changes your life by destroying your dreams? Your own news may be a broken back like Catherine's or the heart attack that forces you off the corporate ladder. It may be the final word that pronounces you infertile and unable to have children to carry your genes. It may be diabetes, with its diet restrictions, possible insulin injections, and the threat of a shortened life span. It may be the word *leukemia* used to describe your twelve-year-old son. It may be the dreaded word *cancer* (that I so often have to pronounce), with all the thoughts of hair loss, nausea, uncontrolled pain, and a shortened life. It may be a hundred other words that forever change the dreams you had for life and open up a world of problems.

What do you do when bad news comes? You have to do something. You have to act to minimize the damage. You have to go on with life. You have to realign your dreams with new boundaries. You have to live in the world as a different person—and live with a God who has acted differently toward you than you expected.

Perhaps you are one who never gave God much thought. If so, you might choose to take such bad news and simply slug it out and fight the battles as a wounded soldier, hoping that the joy in life ahead will be worth the struggle. With family, friends, doctors, and a social system supporting you, you may seek to make life worth living in spite of bad health and broken dreams.

Where does a person's *faith* fit in? Has the question of God's place in your tragedy come to your thoughts yet? Can anyone *really* trust in God when they receive bad news from a doctor?

Perhaps you are a person of faith who suddenly is wondering what difference God is going to make in this crisis. Can those who trust in God make more of life when dreams are shattered than those who live without him? People who trust in God are supposed to be different than those who don't. God's presence is supposed to make that difference—emotionally, spiritually, and physically—when medical tragedy lands in your lap. But can you let your faith enter the complicated arena of medical treatment? Will you let God do his work when *your* doctor hands you bad news? Or will you isolate God's relevance to Sunday mornings and the funeral home?

No matter where we stand in our personal faith, when the doctor brings bad news, most of us *want God to help fix things*. Suddenly our lives have been hit with an earthquake. The world as we know it is trembling, and we are grasping for solid ground. But if we wish to find that stability, our understanding of this world may need to change radically. As the ground continues to shift beneath our feet, perhaps we need to view life differently than before. Perhaps we must grasp a different concept of time, a different notion of reality, a different understanding of value, a different relationship with the Father. Perhaps we must walk in a different Way.

In the Bible, God tells us that death is not the end of life, that life is more than what we touch, that value doesn't have to vanish with tragedy, and that he can provide his presence, peace, purpose, and power in any situation. We've all heard people of faith say that they could walk through any tragedy with God. How then do we do it? Can we grasp this truth that God offers and let it overcome the tragedy we face, or will we bend and break like the world when a doctor tells us that our health will no longer support our dreams? We have choices to make.

When I graduated from high school in 1968, my parents had the foolish courage to allow me and two of my friends to drive to Alaska as a graduation trip. The trip was awesome. Driving that long gravel highway through Canada into the mountains and glaciers of Alaska, we saw the beauty and felt the wonder of life. A fourth friend joined us in Anchorage, and we spent a week touring the state, flying to Nome and Kotzebue, sleeping on stacks of plywood north of the Arctic Circle, swatting mosquitoes bigger than most New York City dogs—a perfect trip for four teenage boys.

My father had loaned us the family station wagon, a black Ford that performed beautifully on that very long and rocky Alcan Highway. One day we were driving in Denali Park, with that great mountain looming before us, and we hit a bump that loosened our teeth. Pretty soon the oil light began to flash, and we discovered a crack in our engine. Prepared for every disaster, we had with us a case of oil in the back of the wagon. Every mile we stopped and poured in another quart. We made it back to Fairbanks but could go no farther; the car was finished. We sold it for fifty dollars and faced the question, "Is this the end of our journey?"

Two interesting decisions were made. One of my buddies' parents said, "Your trip is over. Come home now." He flew directly home from Fairbanks. The rest of us chose to travel home by a different route. It was a difficult journey. We slept in open fields, hitchhiked in the cold night with an old miner and listened to his stories, rode the Alaskan ferry through the beautiful coastal islands, and survived on Ritz crackers with peanut butter.

The journey was hard, but it was one of the best parts of our trip. That bump in Denali Park changed our plans, shortened our trip, and brought extraordinary difficulties to our journey. We, like our friend, could have just given up and flown home. But then we would have missed the relationships, the beauty, and the joy of living that came with that last week of our travels.

Life itself is a great trip for most of us, but there will always come the bump in the road that changes our plans. Each of us, someday, will receive the call or face the doctor who tells us that our dreams are shattered. At that point we will have a choice: will we overcome and live life fully, or will we whimper through the rest of our existence until death? I believe that God did not create us to give up life before he rings the bell. God created us to be overcomers.

Every person has access to all that is necessary to face bad news and broken dreams victoriously.

I have spent more than twenty years of my life caring for suffering people, first as a missionary doctor, then as a medical oncologist. I have often been the doctor handing out the bad news. I have seen many people, both Christians and non-Christians, fall apart and never live again. And I have seen others who, with hope and victory, face the change that bad news brings. I have watched incredible men and women reach down, pick up their broken dreams, and refashion them along God's design into something more beautiful than they had ever been before.

How did they do it so well? Were they unusual people, immune to the trauma of tragedy? Or did they learn something in their walk with God that we too can learn? I believe the latter is true. Every person has access to all that is necessary to face bad news and broken dreams victoriously. God has provided the way. He offers you the freedom to make some powerful choices in the midst of your pain. As you read this book, people who have been there before will point the way, but the choices will be your own.

TWO

Choose God's Place in Your Crisis

EVEN BEFORE CATHERINE HIT THE EMERGENCY ROOM, PEOPLE OF FAITH began to pray to a God whom they believed could help her. Two great pediatric spine doctors took Catherine to the operating room on the morning after her admission and used the best science available to relieve the pressure from her spinal cord and put her spine back together again. One day later Catherine was walking.

As a doctor and father I had chosen the best physicians available. They then used their hard-earned skills and remarkable technology to shift the spine, position titanium rods, set bone grafts, and make my daughter whole again. At the same time we, and people all over the country, were praying fervently to the God we know can heal. Catherine was on her way to health again. Thank God! Thank the doctors!

Who healed Catherine, God or the doctors? What part does science play in our healing, and what part does God play? Is God involved in healing, or is it really only science? Can we trust God to take part in modern medicine, or should we leave him on the sidelines as a most passionate cheerleader? Can we run to God while we are holding the doctor's hand?

EVIDENCE FOR GOD'S HAND IN HEALING

Scientists, too, have wondered whether there is credible evidence that God is involved in healing. The answer is *yes*. There now exist a number of scientific studies in which patients have been randomized to receive only scientific care or scientific care plus prayer. In one such study, patients who were in a coronary-care unit after having a heart attack were randomly assigned to good medical care alone or good medical care plus intercessory prayer by people who believed in God's healing power. Neither the patients nor their doctors knew to which group each was assigned. The results demonstrated a clear improvement in the outcomes of the group covered with prayer. Hundreds of such studies have been gathered and published with more being generated all the time.[1] Science itself now suggests that God plays a role in healing.

Along with the scientific evidence, many of us have personally observed God working to heal. In 1983 God called my family to work as missionaries in Eku, Nigeria. Tim and Janice McCall were close friends and fellow missionaries who lived two houses down in our compound. One night Janice woke us to ask us to come to their house to pray. A poisonous snake had slipped into their house that evening and had bitten their seven-year-old son, David. When we arrived with other missionaries from the compound, David was very ill. He was delirious, and his leg was turning black. There was no antivenom available anywhere in the area. Feeling helplessly dependent on a power greater than our own, we all gathered around David and poured our hearts out before the God who heals. The next morning when we returned to David, his leg was healing, and he was soon completely well.

Both science and personal observation point us to the fact that God heals. For some of us, our own health experience affirms this as well. On about my first birthday my parents noticed that I had become less active and was stagnant in my development. A neurosurgical evaluation revealed that my brain was degenerating and fluid was building up inside my head. My kids still touch the holes in my skull where the doctors attempted to relieve the pressure. Science failed, and my parents were told that I was destined to die or to live my life as a "vegetable." They were told to put me into an institution to decrease the hardship on the rest of my family. My parents refused to give up and instead allowed my Aunt Eunice to take me to her church where faithful Christians laid hands on me and prayed, asking God to heal me. I began to get well and eventually became a doctor who uses science and believes in a God who heals.

Both scientific studies and personal experience provide evidence that points to God's hand in healing, and, though no evidence provides absolute proof, enough exists to make it reasonable to believe that God is involved in the healing process. For many of us who work with science every day, it is very helpful to know that it is reasonable to trust in God for healing.

But suppose we are wrong and science is all there is, where does that alternative lead us? What if human beings are nothing but chemical reactions and biological processes? Ernest Becker, in his book *The Denial of Death*, describes what he calls man's greatest dilemma. Becker says we can dream great dreams, look into the past and imagine we were there, look into the future and see our children's children, gaze at the stars and climb mountain peaks and believe that we are little gods. But in truth, he declares, we are "gods" limited by our biology and "gods who die." In spite of our great imaginations and our desire to become heroes, we are really only animals, limited by a body that breaks and a future in which we are food for worms.

For many who work with science, it is helpful to know that it is reasonable to trust in God for healing.

Becker writes that human beings are unable to face this dilemma and live sanely. To protect our sanity, we set up complex psychological barriers, then live as if we cannot die. Unable to accept God's involvement in our lives, we are stuck with the knowledge that our lives are left to the processes of a natural world. We then close our eyes to the brokenness and death that a natural world brings. When nature works against us, we depend on science as our only hope.[2]

Is this an acceptable alternative for you? Or would you rather believe in a God who actively cares for your life and health?

Based on all these considerations, I, as a doctor, choose to believe that God is involved in healing, and I choose to do so for three reasons:

1. The evidence is consistent.
2. The alternative is unacceptable.
3. And most important, I have a relationship with, and have learned to trust, the God who heals.

Suppose I am right and God *is* involved in healing. As I watched Catherine's event unfold, and as you look at your own health circumstances, where can we actually see God at work? Let me lay one more foundation stone for you to consider, and then I'll list the ways that I can see God active in injury or illness.

Health Is God's Invention

Though most of us think of health as normal and unremarkable, health, in truth, is awesome. As Michael Behe describes in his book *Darwin's Black Box,* our bodies are so complex that it would be mathematically impossible for us to exist by accidental evolution. Good science demands a Designer behind our ongoing existence. For example, in order for our blood to clot properly when we are cut, many things must happen at the same time. Cell fragments called platelets move in to plug the leak; then proteins form a clot around the platelets. In order for this clot to form, at least thirteen proteins in two parallel systems must react with each other in the proper sequence. This sequential reaction of proteins initiates another system, which places the brakes on the clot so it doesn't go too far. At the same time, another system is triggered to dissolve any excessive clot. An error in any one part of any of these systems could lead to a person's bleeding or clotting to death. This incredible balance goes on constantly throughout our lives with every little nick and bump, and rarely does it fail us.[3]

Take cancer as another example. Cancer is a disease that starts within our DNA. Mutations within our genetic code in a single cell allow that cell to divide and escape the body's normal regulatory systems, thus forming a cancerous growth. Were you aware that every day, mutations are occurring in our cells that could turn into cancers?

Yet most of us don't suffer from cancer. That's because our great Designer has placed within our cells special mechanisms to sniff out mistakes in our genes as they happen and correct them, preventing most cancers from ever developing.

When I look at these complex biological systems that make up who I am, I realize that health doesn't just happen by accident. *Health is God's invention and could not exist without God's control*. If this is true, there must follow another truth about scientific medicine: when we discover new things about the body through science, we are uncovering truths that have been placed there by God. The discovery of scientific truth is an uncovering of God's truth.

The discovery of scientific truth is an uncovering of God's truth.

GOD'S WORK IN HEALING

With this foundation, let me list eight ways that God is involved in healing:

1. God maintains our health through design. It amazes me that my daughter Catherine was able to perform aggressive gymnastics for nine years without breaking her back until now. It was God's incredible design of nerves, muscles, and bones, and his constant maintenance that allowed her to fly through the air and land on her feet time and time again. Though your body may be broken now, it has served you well in a miraculous way in the past and will continue to do so in many ways, even with the changes ahead of you.

2. God protects our health through moral instruction. How many diseases would never kill? How many traumas would never maim if we followed God's instructions in the Bible? God created us because he loves us, and he did not leave us without instructions to protect us from a difficult world. There are lessons we can learn from his Word that will serve us well in our future health.

3. God reveals scientific knowledge and develops our skills to use it. The two doctors who worked on Catherine's spine studied and practiced for years to gain the necessary knowledge and skills to mend her brokenness. The truth they discovered about broken spines during those long years of study was God's truth, about God's creation, revealed to mankind to relieve suffering. The minds and dexterity that transformed that truth into effective action were given to these doctors as a gift from God. This same scientific knowledge and skill are available to you as you face an illness that needs mending.

4. God is present in power. God was present in that surgical suite with those doctors and Catherine because God loved them, because he had a plan for their lives, and because of our faith. When I saw Catherine walk again, there flashed into my mind one of my favorite Scripture passages: "He took her by the hand and said to her, '*Talitha koum!*' (which means, 'Little girl, I say to you get up!'). Immediately the girl stood up and walked around (she was twelve years old)" (Mark 5:41–42).

That passage has now been brought to life for me by the power of God working through the actions of these doctors. God not only provides the science, he is present in power as that science is used. There are great questions regarding God's power that we will deal with later, but I assure you, God's power is the ultimate source of all healing.

5. God listens to the prayers of his followers. Catherine did not face her injury alone. As Catherine's spine shifted when she fell, it moved backward to crush her spinal cord, but then it stopped one millimeter short. God's power, as he held back the bones of the spine from moving that last millimeter and as he worked through the hands of Catherine's surgeons, was somehow facilitated by the hundreds of people praying for Catherine's healing. It is an awesome and mysterious responsibility God hands his followers: to direct his power, within his will, through our prayers of faith.

Earlier this month I placed my hand on the shoulder of a forty-seven-year-old woman with cancer. I knew that science said, "She cannot be healed." Nevertheless I prayed to God that he would heal her completely. This woman knew the truth of her illness, but I made certain she also understood the truth of God's power. Every week one or two patients out of a hundred walk into my office healthy, after science had told them, "You cannot be healed." Through great prayer and God's power these patients stand before me, underlining the truth that God is indeed greater than the science he created.

6. God blesses illness with purpose. As Catherine was recovering, my mother revealed to us her feelings of guilt over Catherine's injury. Before the accident, because of her gymnastics Catherine had developed few friends, had little interest in school, and showed minimal concern for the church. Her grandmother had prayed for God to change Catherine's life so that she might grow up whole and happy. When the injury came, with its near paralysis and prolonged recovery, Catherine's grandmother felt responsible and guilty because of her prayers. In truth, Catherine is now a well-balanced scholar, is active in three high school sports, attends church regularly, and has never been happier. I do not know whether God worked to cause Catherine's injury, but he did work to produce out of that injury a very good result.

God brings purpose to illness and injury, where otherwise there might be only tragedy. It may not be clear to you what good can come of an injury or illness when you first receive the doctor's bad news, but it is always clear to God. He will not waste your suffering. Some good will come from it.

7. God blesses illness with peace. I often see a great fear or anxiety in my patients when I tell them they have cancer and might die, but that is not always the case. A Christian ophthalmologist named James Collier developed lung cancer that would eventually spread throughout his body and take his life. In the middle of his journey through that terrible illness, he wrote, "I know Jesus is all I have and all I need. I've learned to live in the joy of the moment. I've learned to practice the presence of God. . . . I know where the road ends. I don't know how much longer my journey will be. But I do know His majesty awaits me at the end of the road. I can tell you from the bottom of my heart that I would not trade the trip for anything. I would not take away the cancer if it meant missing the journey into the deeper waters of God's love. It has been wonderful."[4]

As a cancer physician, I have had patient after patient tell me that God has brought them such incredible peace within their illness that it made it worth having the illness for the peace they have gained. How can we help make your experience with illness become the same? I pray that the pages of this book hold part of the answer.

8. God completes our health in heaven. God often demonstrates his power through science. He sometimes demonstrates his power *around* science to heal those who are ill or injured. But any healing we witness on earth is temporary. Even Lazarus died again, and when he died, it seemed as but a blink of an eye since Jesus had raised him from the dead. The only healing on this earth that is permanent is that which transforms our temporary bodies into eternal ones.

Oscar Arnulfo Romero was the archbishop of San Salvador in the 1970s during a time of great political upheaval. He fought for the poor and the oppressed. One day he said in an interview, "I have frequently been threatened with death. I must say that, as a Christian, I do not believe in *death*, but in the *resurrection*." Two weeks later, as he was saying mass in the chapel of a cancer hospital, he was shot and killed for living out his faith.[5] As a Christian, Oscar Romero had anticipated a life with God after his life on earth was over. He therefore lived passionately and without fear because of that anticipation. Whatever our illness or injury, when we call ourselves Christians, we are counting on a day ahead, through God's grace and God's power, when we too will experience perfect healing as we are raised from death into a perfect life with God and with our loved ones.

Now that the doctor has delivered the bad news to you, does God have a place in your healing? If you are forced to live this life with illness, without a miracle or scientific cure, will God be walking with you?

Each of us must decide for ourselves. Your illness or tragedy, whatever it is, is giving you the chance to address this question now. I am writing this book because I know there is a critical choice to be made. If you choose to place your hand in God's hand, like James Collier and many others I have known, you will be able to walk your difficult road in peace. Perhaps, like some of them, in spite of your illness, you may even call your life *wonderful*.

A few years ago I had the privilege of listening to Drs. Paul and Margaret Brand as they spoke to a gathering of Christian physicians. Dr. Margaret Brand, a great missionary doctor who worked alongside her husband for years in the leper colonies of India and in Louisiana, told the story of a brilliant young Indian man with an engineering degree who could speak four languages and was soon to be married. Then he contracted tuberculosis and leprosy. He lost his bride, lost his job, and would someday lose his life to the diseases. He stayed at the leprosy hospital for many months. It was a Christian hospital, but whenever Dr. Brand spoke to the young man about God's love, he became angry and said, "God took away from me everything I loved."

A nurse's aide named David worked on the ward and did his work with constant joy. Somehow this joy was a salve for the young engineer, and one day David led the engineer to know Christ. There was an immediate transformation. This bitter, defeated young man became a man with joy in his heart and on his tongue. Joy remained with him for the rest of his life. One day, with his tuberculosis progressing, it was necessary for him to have a lung removed. It was very serious surgery from which he might die. Before his surgery, this transformed engineer said, "Why should I be afraid? If I die, I go to be with Jesus; if I live, he is here with me." He lived another six months. Just prior to his death he wrote a letter to Dr. Brand that said, "I am glad that I caught leprosy, for with it I found God."

Whether the doctor's bad news will shorten your life or just make it more difficult, God promises to work in your illness. Much of the peace you seek within your difficult circumstances can be found if you walk in the presence of God, with the knowledge that he is there with both love and power.

> Though the fig tree does not bud
> and there are no grapes on the vines,
> though the olive crop fails
> and the fields produce no food,
> though there are no sheep in the pen
> and no cattle in the stalls,
> yet I will rejoice in the Lord,
> I will be joyful in God my Savior.
>
> —HABAKKUK 3:17–18

THREE

Choose the Best Science

Michael was young and handsome. His wife was attractive and attentive with intelligent eyes. When I greeted them in the examining room, they both appeared quite healthy and normal. But Michael had had a brain tumor, discovered after he had developed headaches. The tumor had been removed surgically. His only complaint now was that an area of his vision was missing. He and his wife had come to me for advice regarding further therapy. I interviewed Michael, examined him, then explained my understanding of his situation.

"You have a glioblastoma, Michael. That's a malignant brain tumor. Your surgeon has done a good job of removing it all, but there's a very high probability it will return. I recommend that we do our best to delay its return with radiation therapy and some new oral chemotherapy, but I don't believe we will be able it cure it forever."

Michael and Robin took the news stoically and returned later with a number of questions.

"How long can I live?"

"Where should we go for any new research treatments?"

"What do you think about this information we found on the internet?"

"What do you think about shark cartilage?"

I took their questions one at a time and worked through them. We developed a final plan for Michael to visit the Brain Tumor Clinic at Duke University for an experimental therapy that looked hopeful.

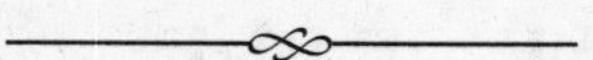

What do you do when the doctor first tells you bad news? The bad news might be a malignancy, like Michael's, or it could be infertility, multiple sclerosis, diabetes, a debilitating injury, heart disease, or any of a number of other diagnoses that halt your rush through life with the realization that your life has changed in a tragic way.

It has been my experience that a blanket of shock settles over patients when they first hear the bad news. They understand very little else I say at that visit and leave in somewhat of a daze. Hearing the bad news is the first step on a long and difficult journey, and it is often a step taken in the fog.

Many questions need to be asked and answered for patients so they can be certain they are receiving the best possible medical care. Let me list for you the ones I feel are important. Don't try to ask these questions when you first are told the bad news. If time allows, make another appointment with your doctor as soon as possible. I recommend you bring a support person with you to help you clarify issues. And carry either a notepad or tape recorder to help you remember and understand the doctor's answers and advice.

Questions for the Doctor

1. How confident are you of the diagnosis? Sometimes doctors are absolutely certain about the diagnosis, but sometimes we're not. Sometimes a different problem might mimic your diagnosis. And sometimes the consequences of an abnormality may not be as grave as a doctor assumes. Patients should understand the level of confidence a doctor has in the diagnosis and whether it would be worthwhile to perform other studies to verify it.

One young man I am still following had testicular cancer a few years ago. We treated him appropriately. One year later his chest X ray showed nodules that were almost certainly cancer metastases (cancer that spread from the original site). However, even a 90 percent probability was inadequate in his case, so I biopsied the nodules, finding instead a very treatable histoplasmosis in his lungs. Be certain, as a patient, that you know the level of confidence your doctor has in your diagnosis.

2. What will this problem do to the length and quality of my life? You must understand your illness in order to choose the best possible therapeutic approach and to plan your life realistically. A seventy-one-year-old man, previously healthy, developed multiple myeloma. Myeloma is a malignancy of the bone marrow that dissolves the bony tissue, leaving holes and causing fractures. His question of chief importance was, "Can you get me back on the golf course, Doc?" That was his important quality-of-life issue. My answer was, "I'm not sure we can, but we will try our best to get you there and let you know as soon as we are certain." For other folks it's not golf but tennis or violin or even reading a book. The more you as a patient can understand the disease or condition you are facing and how it will affect the quality of your life, the better you can adjust your physical, social, and business life around it. We will discuss more about your quality of life in a later chapter.

"How long will I live?" The doctor is rarely able to give precise answers to this question at first. There is tremendous variability from patient to patient in every disease process. When you are given an estimate, realize that you are listening to that doctor's knowledge of *average* cases. Ask, "What is the best I could possibly hope for?" and "What is the worst I could anticipate happening?" You probably are somewhere within that range.

3. What is the best treatment for my problem? When I see a patient, there are always three possible goals to therapy. The first would be to *cure the problem.* If this is not medically possible, the second would be to *help the patient live as long as possible.* The third goal is always operative and sometimes the only possible goal: to *insure that the quality of life of my patient is the best it can be.* Sometimes one goal is paramount;

sometimes another is. I must be very clear about the goals when I suggest therapy. If I'm not clear, my patient may become lost in the maze of medical science with a great deal of cost and trouble but very little real benefit. When my patient understands the best and most appropriate goal of therapy, that patient can then decide whether the cost and difficulty of therapy are worthwhile. Your doctor should explain the treatment, tell you which goals can be accomplished, and inform you whether there are other options to reach those goals. Ask the doctor for written information about your illness. You should receive information prepared for patients or an internet site that will help you better understand your problem. But be careful about exploring the internet without guidance. Anyone can put information on the internet, and many do so with misguided motives. Ask your doctor for reliable internet sites to help you research your problem. Keep in mind: treatment that doesn't meet any of the three listed goals is of little value, even if the condition improves for a while.

4. Should I seek a second opinion? It is always okay to ask this question. Anyone who is faced with a life-changing health problem should hear the diagnosis from at least two doctors, or from one doctor whom that patient trusts completely. Based on your confidence in the doctor and your confidence in the answer, decide whether a second opinion is warranted. If you are seeing a specialist regarding your problem, always discuss his information with your primary doctor to get a different level of interpretation. Ask your primary doctor to help you decide whether a second opinion would be worth the cost and trouble. If you decide to forgo a second opinion, be sure you are willing to accept the results of your treatment without looking back at this question with regret.

5. Are there any research programs in which I should consider taking part? Sometimes a research therapy is the best hope for a terrible medical problem. At other times research trials are very difficult and offer little hope of benefit. Don't trust your aunt, uncle, cousin, or the internet regarding the benefits of research. Ask your doctor to explore research possibilities and tell you which ones might be worth the trouble they bring in travel, cost, discomfort, or sickness. Most doctors want only the best for their patients and are happy to refer them for research trials that offer real hope. Some research trials, in fact, are the best hope for a patient's well-being. Remember: Any research program proven to be better than standard treatment would no longer be experimental. Your doctor probably is the best one to judge whether a research trial is more likely to help you than usual therapy.

6. What about alternative and complementary medicines? Many people, when they are faced with serious health problems, use alternative and complementary medicines and therapies. Some use them in addition to the doctor's medical care, while others choose alternative therapies as a substitute for standard medical care. I am still heartbroken over a young woman who came to me after an operation for very treatable cancer. After our discussions, she decided instead to visit a holistic medicine clinic that focused on enemas and nutrition to maximize the immune system. When she returned with advanced cancer, it was too late to provide her any real hope of a cure.

There is no adequate testing for most alternative medicines to understand side effects or interactions with standard treatments.

More commonly, patients keep quiet about their alternative medicines and use them silently while also taking the treatment offered by the doctor. There are two major problems with alternative medicines. The first is their lack of proven effectiveness. Standard medicines undergo rigorous trials to be certain they are effective. Any standard medicine has clearly recorded information regarding the percentage of people who might benefit from its use. There is no such reliable information for alternative medicines. The other problem with alternative therapies is an inadequate understanding of their toxicities. There is no adequate testing for most alternative medicines to understand either their side effects or their interactions with standard treatments. No one knows whether most alternative therapies will help or interfere with your doctor's treatment for your medical problem.

I don't doubt that many alternative therapies are potent, and some may produce benefits in some patients. Medical doctors recognize this, and studies are under way to test these therapies for effectiveness and toxicities. Worthwhile information is already available for some alternative therapies. One excellent reference is *Alternative Medicine: The Christian Handbook* by Donal O'Mathuna and Walt Larimore.[1] Ask your doctor specifically about any alternative therapies that you might like to try and let him or her research it for you.

7. Doctor, if I were your mother, what would you tell me to do? In the last twenty years, decision-making in American medicine has been handed over to the patient. American doctors in general want their patients to make the decisions regarding their therapy after fully informing them of the therapeutic options, the risks, and the potential benefits. Sometimes all of this information leaves the patient anxious and unable to make a decision. It is usually appropriate to ask the doctor which of the options would be the doctor's choice for one of his or her family members. Make it a personal decision for the doctor.

An eighty-year-old woman came to me with lung cancer that had spread to her liver. She was weak but not in pain. I explained to her the option of chemotherapy as an aggressive attempt to treat her cancer. I also explained the option of hospice care with no treatment of the cancer, but supportive care to keep her as active and comfortable through the final stages of her disease. I did not tell her what to do. She looked me in the eyes and asked me, "What would you tell your mother to do?" I answered with both my head and my heart. "If you were my mother, I would tell you to leave the treatment alone and to get the most you can out of every day left in your life without us giving you all this stuff to make you sick." She smiled and turned to her children. "That's what I want." Consider asking your doctor the same question. If a doctor refuses to answer this question, there may be a problem either with the doctor's level of commitment to you or in the confidence the doctor has in some of the options.

8. Do you pray with your patients, doctor? When you are struck with terrible medical news, the rest of your illness will be easier to bear if your doctor will pray with you. There are many benefits of praying with your doctor.

- Prayer invites God into your health-care process so that the power of science and the power of God can work together toward your healing.
- Your doctor will become more committed to you on a personal level.
- Your doctor will understand the importance of your faith in your life and will feel more open to discuss spiritual matters with you in the future.
- Your doctor will be blessed personally by that encounter with the Creator.

As you think about the bad news you have received, you probably will have other questions. Some of these might be:

> "How urgent is treatment? I've got some things I need to do."
>
> "What about my children? Is this inherited? How can I help them deal with my illness?"
>
> "What is the cost of treatment?"
>
> "Do you know of support groups for counseling in which I can participate?"
>
> "What kind of activity may I continue?"
>
> "Should I be on any special diet?"

All of these are common questions, and the answers may be helpful. You should ask the first eight I have listed at some time early in the course of your illness or injury, then add others as appropriate for you.

When you are faced with life-changing bad news, part of your suffering is the fear of not knowing. There is always some degree of uncertainty in every life-changing event, but with proper and complete information, that uncertainty can be minimized. You can then use this information to plan your most hopeful course of therapy and your best pathway to complete the life that God has called you to live. With those decisions made, you can take the time you would have spent wringing your hands and instead use it to hold hands with a loved one, to laugh with the kids, to lift up others who are broken, and to thank God for the good things of life.

[illegible]

[illegible] gradual weight gain.

[illegible]

[illegible]

Your [illegible] will [illegible]

[illegible]

As [illegible]

How long [illegible]

What about [illegible] How will [illegible]

What is the cost of treatment?

[illegible]

What kind of [illegible]

[illegible]

[illegible]

FOUR

Choose Reality

Do we really understand what life is all about, or do we settle for only half of reality?

The last time I was in Albania, helping to revive a wounded health-care system, I heard the true story of a young doctor I will call Anton. Anton had been an atheist until six years before. Prior to the event I am describing, he and his wife were childless, having suffered three miscarriages. Finally a new pregnancy filled their lives with hope. But in the tragedy of another miscarriage, that hope died, and Anton held a tiny, dead child in his hand. He and his wife scheduled a surgical procedure for the next day to clean out her wasted womb. That night Anton was on call and slept at the hospital. In a dream a very old woman came to him and offered him two medallions—one gold and one silver. Anton refused to take such a gift from a patient in spite of her repeated insistence. In that dream, Anton fell asleep. He awoke, still in the dream, to find the old woman gone and the medallions left behind on his bed. When Anton really awakened the next morning, he was troubled by his dream and told the story of the old lady and the medallions to his mother-in law, who was a very religious woman. Anton's mother-in-law listened and interpreted the dream. The old woman in the dream, she said, was a messenger from God, bringing him two

Christian medallions. She had come to promise Anton that he would have a child, a son. Now, Anton knew this was impossible; he had held the dead fetus in his hands. But Anton was so troubled by the dream that he insisted on an ultrasound before his wife's surgery. His wife's doctor while watching the ultrasound cried out, "There is a child!"

Anton's wife was still bleeding from the miscarriage, so for five months she remained in bed. Finally Anton's wife bore them a healthy son. The boy was born on Christmas day, so his parents named him Christie. With that birth Anton began to believe in God and has loved him ever since.

As you face the tragic news of broken health, how small is your world? Will you settle for only the concrete and the visible? Could reality encompass a spiritual world beyond your senses? How limited is your spirit? How confined is your understanding of reality?

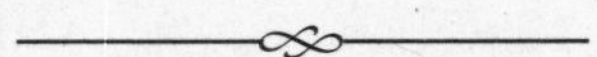

Mrs. Mallery died from a sarcoma that filled her lungs. The day after her death her husband told me about her last two days. On the day before she died, she had been somewhat confused from her pain medicines. But there came a time of full mental clarity, and she told her daughter, "I saw God today."

The daughter responded, "Did you really? Were his angels with him?"

Mrs. Mallery replied, "Yes, they were, and they are coming soon for me. But I told them they had to wait just a bit longer because you and Daddy still needed me."

The next day Mrs. Mallery died. When the daughter started to weep, her father said, "Don't cry. This is beautiful. She is with God, just where she has always wanted to be."

Did Mrs. Mallery really see God? Is there anything to this life beyond what we can see, touch, taste, hear, and prove with mathematics or a microscope? Is there really something more than the material world to help me when the doctor delivers bad news?

Rachel was our friend. She was thirty years old, had a beautiful Nigerian smile, and carried our daughter Catherine on her back wherever she went in the village of Eku. As the *juju* festival was approaching, we asked her about these spirits of the forest that townspeople worshiped. She told of the *adada*—children who were destined to serve the *juju* as priestesses. They can be identified, she explained, by the way their hair curls as it grows. Once the priests choose them, they may never cut their hair or they will be killed. Rachel also told us how the river *juju* would claim one life each year from the village as a sacrifice. That year a young boy had drowned in the beautiful Ethiope River that ran near our house. I asked Rachel whether she was afraid to be surrounded by such spirits. She grinned and said, "They cannot harm me. I am a Christian!" Rachel had no difficulty in accepting a spiritual world beyond our senses and fitting that world into her everyday life.

SCIENCE AND REALITY

In our modern society we tend to believe only those things we can touch or test. We call that science. But perhaps we have given science too much responsibility. Scientific thinking is certainly of great value to us, but we err if we separate science from God. Science comes from God. Scientific thinking is a God-given tool to help us handle problems in this world of ours. There is no more conflict between God and science than there is between a gardener and a shovel. If God is the Creator of all things, whatever we discover in science is God's truth. From the discovery of the wheel to the newest techniques in reproductive technology, God knew it first; God designed it before we were born, then handed this knowledge to us as a means to ease the suffering of those we love. Galileo knew this. When Galileo proved scientifically that the earth revolved around the sun, he was persecuted by the church because Galileo's science at that time did not agree with the church's understanding of theology. But Galileo personally had no problem accepting fully the authority of God's Word and, at the same time, using science for what it offered. He felt that no two truths could contradict each other, so someday, this scientific truth and the Bible would become, of necessity, perfectly harmonious.[1]

Galileo understood that science is a long way from discovering all truth, but when science is done well, it will eventually confirm the rightful place of God the Creator. Scientific truth is imperfect because there is so much out there yet to learn. But, imperfect as it is, God's knowledge, through science, is handed to God's doctors to help overcome the problems in this world that break down our bodies.

The problem that we as people of faith have with science is the responsibility we have laid upon it. In modern society we have expanded the responsibility of science to let it be the definer of reality. We have changed the statement "reality is what is" to "reality is what I can prove."

This is simply not true. Science is too incomplete to define reality. Newly discovered facts continually change our theories and bring to us new understandings of reality. For example, on three occasions during my time in Nigeria, patients were brought to me with terribly burned feet. Each had a history of a seizure disorder. When asked about the feet, the families would explain, "He done die. We place his feet in the fire, and he done get life again." Some local tribesman must have once observed people who had had seizures, then fell to the ground as if dead but noticed that some who had fallen into the fire came back to life. From this observation, in rural Nigeria they developed the theory that people who died after a seizure might be brought back to life if their feet were placed in the fire. The theory was tested, and a few of the "dead" came back to life (those who had had seizures and only looked dead). Since the test sometimes confirmed the theory, the villagers acted upon the theory. Henceforth when anyone who had a seizure became unconscious, villagers would place their feet into a fire.

Science is a long way from discovering all truth, but it will eventually confirm the rightful place of God the Creator.

Now new knowledge has come. Nigerian physicians have now learned medical knowledge that is unknown to many of the villagers. They have learned about brain waves and electrical short circuits and EEGs, and they know that seizure patients often look dead after a grand mal seizure but will wake up and be fine, fire or no fire. Reality for Nigerian villagers, based on what they could touch and see, is "Fire can give life." With new facts available, reality for Nigerian physicians has become, "Fire burns feet and has nothing to do with restoring life to seizure patients." The new knowledge has changed what educated Nigerians believe is reality. What was reality based on observation changed when new information was revealed.

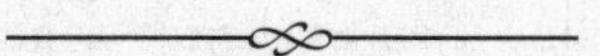

We, too, have incomplete knowledge and should not, therefore, allow science to define the limits of reality. Our tendency is to assume that those things we cannot prove must not exist. This has never been an assumption of true science, but it has nevertheless made its way into modern people's understanding of life in the name of science. If we can prove it, it is true. If we cannot prove it, it is not true. That kind of thinking is faulty. Throughout history, theories that intelligent people swore were false were proven later to be true when tools were developed to provide the proof. Galileo was sentenced to life in prison because he theorized the earth revolved around the sun before he had the instruments to prove it. We use science to help prove that our theories are true, but it is illogical to believe that our inability to prove something confirms that it does not exist. Our lack of proof may simply result from our lack of adequate knowledge or tools to resolve the question at that time. Science is useful to explore our world, but it should never define the limits of our reality.

What has this to do with how you face illness? If, when facing illness, the only reality you can accept is that which can be touched and tested through science, then that limits your hope. But we who believe in God know that science is incomplete, and we know there is a reality beyond that which can be tested by scientific means. Scientific thinking has not yet found the tools to test the existence of the spiritual world, so many people have assumed it cannot exist. But life does have a spiritual dimension whether or not science can ever prove it.

I was traveling with David Egbedion to his church in Ughere, Nigeria, for a Thanksgiving service. On the way, he told me of a woman in his church who had miscarried six babies at six to seven months gestation and thus had no children. She dreamed at night of evil spirits and became certain they were preventing her from having a child. Offerings by her husband to various *jujus* had not helped.

David explained to her that God was stronger than those spirits. If she accepted Jesus as her Savior, they would have no power over her. She did accept Jesus, and from that moment she saw no more evil spirits and has had two babies with no miscarriages. No scientist can prove the presence of this woman's evil spirits, and many scientists would doubt them, but their existence is at least as plausible as a sudden random change in fertility.

You need not personally accept the existence of evil spirits, but you will never find hope beyond science and hope beyond death if you do not accept a spiritual dimension to reality. There must be more to life than matter. The Egyptian pharaohs were mummified so their bodies would last forever. Their bodies can be touched today as they were three thousand years ago, but that was not the point of their mummification. The pharaohs had their bodies mummified because they believed in an afterworld where their *spirit* would rejoin their *matter*. As far as I'm concerned, if our world is only matter, and I'm dead forever when my body quits working, I couldn't care less how long my tissue is preserved. If matter is all there is, is it really very important whether I have to take insulin shots or cardiac drugs or chemotherapy for the few remaining years that my body functions? At some time in our lives, all of us long for another plane of life, beyond our five senses, that is just as real, that can make our short lives more significant.

There was a day in history when a city in the small kingdom of Israel was surrounded by the army of Aram (2 Kings 6:8–17). Reading that story, I wonder what it would feel like to wake up with my city surrounded by an enemy planning to destroy me. Perhaps not much different than the way we feel when face-to-face with bad news from our doctor.

When the Israelites looked out from the city, they saw thousands of soldiers and chariots poised to attack. But there was more to see than what the Israelites saw. Elisha's eyes saw more, and when he prayed, his servant saw the same. Surrounding the army of destruction was the Lord's great army, ready to fight against the forces of Aram.

What was the difference between Elisha's eyes and the eyes of the Israelites? Elisha saw more than that which could be grasped by his five senses. Elisha looked with eyes of faith and, in doing so, saw the realm of the spirit, just as real and alive as the physical realm—real and alive enough to destroy the army of Aram.

Do you believe only in the visible as you face your illness? You have the choice in this life to say, "What I see is all there is," and then live it until it ends that way, or you can say with your life, "I believe there is more than that: God is real. He is with me though I cannot see him. He has the power and desire to act in my life to accomplish great things, including the destruction of the army that surrounds me with illness and death."

Life is spirit just as much as it is matter. We can know that only if we view the world through eyes like Elisha's, the eyes of faith. There is a poignant moment in the movie *The Santa Clause* when the business executive who inadvertently took on the job of Santa Claus views the extraordinary North Pole complex with all of its elves and toys. He turns to his thousand-year-old elf hostess and says, "I see it, but I don't believe it!" She answers, "Seeing is not believing; believing is seeing."[2] For some divine reason, God has created us in such a way that the more we trust him, the more we see him at work in our lives. We must believe that God *will* work in our lives in order to *see* God work.

There is one additional step to take toward seeing God work in our difficulties. As we approach a life with wounded health, we may accept the importance of belief in God and even force ourselves to believe that God is there for us, but we still might fail to find the peace we are seeking. God has insisted that the eyes of faith require more than simple belief; the eyes of faith must be *clarified* by real trust. Ron Lively, a former regional director for the Christian Medical and Dental Society, once described a family conference he directed. The children attending the conference were blindfolded in a big room filled with dozens of parents. The parents began to call out their children's names, all at once. In the midst of the din, the children would listen for the voice of their parents, go to that voice blindfolded, and then fall back into the arms belonging to the voice they trusted.

As you are surrounded by circumstances that will cause you great pain or despair and are blindfolded by the nature of the world, are you willing to listen for the voice of God and practice falling into his arms? Only after you have fallen into the arms of God can the blindfold be removed and you finally see with your eyes what you have trusted in your heart.

Life without God is like walking through a great room painted by Michelangelo—with all the lights off. All the beauty is there, but you cannot see it. You come to the end of the room and slide to the ground. You don't know that two feet away there is a door leading to another room—with lights on, with more walls painted by Michelangelo, walls that go on forever. And what is worse, there is a switch to turn on the lights in the room where you now sit. If you had only known you could have turned on the lights and enjoyed the beauty of the room. If you had only reached up and touched the switch (see Matt. 9:21).

The Question of Time

Part of the reason we misunderstand reality is that we misunderstand time. When I first arrived in Nigeria as a missionary, one of my most difficult adjustments came in adapting to the Nigerian concept of time. There would be a meeting scheduled to start at nine, and I would arrive at nine o'clock to find no one there. Nine was the time the Nigerians began thinking about going to the meeting. They would eventually trickle in, with the meeting starting an hour or so later. I would attend church with my Nigerian friends, already having planned a Sunday afternoon with my wife and daughters, only to discover there was no definite ending time for the service. My timed plans with my family would just fade into the late afternoon. There was a difference in Nigerian time and American time. If I had persisted with my American notion of time while living within the Nigerian culture, I would have remained frustrated and angry throughout my two years there.

There is also a difference between human time and God's time. With human time we see life as an experience confined between the boundaries of birth and death. With God's time life goes on forever. God's time does not end with death. You may be facing an illness that threatens to shorten your life. If you hold on to a human understanding of time when death approaches, you may well feel angry and without hope. But with God's understanding of time you can anticipate death as a blessing rather than a curse.

I recently received a letter from the husband of a patient who had died. Both of them loved the Lord and believed in an eternal duration of life. As he spoke of his departed wife, he said: "I sincerely believe that God needed another angel, so he came and took Marion home. Her illness was a means in which to teach me and anyone else who knew her the true definition of faith in God, courage, hope, and love. . . . She constantly said that God truly blessed her. I love and miss her very much. There is a deep, black hole that hurts very much where my heart was. But you and I must remember, there is a new angel in heaven, glorifying our Lord and Savior and watching over you and me." This dear woman, as she was dying, and her husband, after her death, carried a great peace in their hearts, knowing that time does not end with death but continues into eternity with the God who created and loves us.

Jesus described this eternal life when he spoke to the woman at the well in Samaria. Before she met Jesus, the woman probably saw time as a narrow space in the heat of the day when she could fetch water without other women—respectable women—looking askance and whispering about her. Before meeting Jesus, she probably thought of time as that which separated one failed relationship from another. She was not only thirsty for water, she was thirsty for acceptance and a relationship that would last. Then she met Jesus, who said, "If you continue drinking this water, you will thirst again, but if you drink the water I give you, you will never be thirsty. Indeed, the water I give you will become in you a spring of water welling up to eternal life" (John 4:13–14, my paraphrase).

If you believe life goes on forever, you think about death not as the end of life but as the beginning of eternal life.

Jesus was speaking of not only a new quality in life here on earth but also a new duration of life with eternity as its limit. If you believe life is confined between birth and death, then you see death as the end. But if you believe life goes on forever, you think about death not as the end of life but as the beginning of eternal life.

Our hope for heaven does not diminish the importance of our time on earth. How long we live on this side of heaven is certainly important to us, but there is more to our time on earth than its length. When we look at our life, the timing of our death, and the brevity of it all, no matter how long we live, we come to realize that the value of time lies not only in how long life lasts but in how we use each day. Time is not a line that begins with birth and ends with death nor even a line that extends on through death into eternity. Time is more like an Impressionist painting in which each day God paints the picture of our life with multicolored dots. Each colored dot is filled with opportunity. As time passes, the portrait grows. Each dot is separate, but all the dots, seen together, form a picture of our life that is never finished. Death is another dot—black for some, golden for others—and the dots continue. The value of our lives must not be in the number of dots but in the beauty within each dot and in the way each dot adds to the total picture of our life. As we live, and especially as we contemplate death, we must live each day to make each dot as beautiful as possible. Too many of us worry so much about tomorrow that we pass through today without even realizing that it happened. We must recognize and appreciate the joy in each day, even near the end of life.

> *The value of time lies not only in how long life lasts but in how we use each day.*

I like the way my previous pastor, Earl Davis, articulates how we value life: "We go through this life filling our pockets with gold and our hearts with trash, racing ahead, glancing over our shoulders because death is gaining on us." We must realize that the true value of life is not in a future that eludes us or in a past that haunts us, not in our hopes or dreams but within each day as we live it.

Emily knew this. She had advanced bilateral breast cancer when I met her. The treatment we provided made her quite ill for many months and left her with residual heart damage. She is now in remission from her cancer and this past year sat on the end of my examining table and told me, "It is amazing how this illness has changed my life for the better."

"Tell me," I said.

"It has made me so appreciative of each day and what I have—even days when I am suffering. It has improved my prayer life tremendously. It has made my husband and me care for each other so much more."

In her suffering, Emily discovered the significance of each day. No day is empty and meaningless if we choose to fill it, for there are relationships worth eternity in every day we live. As God tells us in his Word, worrying about the future does little to change the future because it is worry based on uncertainty. There is one certainty about our future that each one of us can know: God will be there with us, and he is the God whose "heart is kind beyond all measure." We can trust this one who holds our future, for his only motivation is love.

No day is empty if we choose to fill it, for there are relationships worth eternity in every day we live.

In her book *The Hiding Place,* Corrie ten Boom tells of her imprisonment in Nazi concentration camps with her sister, both sent there for hiding Jews from the Nazi exterminators. As she faced death daily, Corrie remembered back to the time when she was a little girl and cried to her father, "I need you! You can't die! You can't!" Recognizing her fear of death at the time, her father asked her, "Corrie, when you and I go to Amsterdam, when do I give you the ticket?"

"Why, just before we get on the train."

"Exactly. And our wise Father in heaven knows when we're going to need things, too. Don't run out ahead of Him, Corrie. When the time comes that some of us will have to die, you will look into your heart and find the strength you need—just in time."[3]

The Giver of life knows what we need and when we need it. Though we face life with impatience and death with fear, we can trust in his timing and know with certainty that he will be there when the time is right to show us his character of kindness and love.

For every one of us, life on this earth is short. None of us knows when our life will end. For some, the end of this present life is visible, like the dark entrance to a tunnel one hundred yards ahead. For the rest of us, that tunnel is around one or two more bends in the mountains. Either way, if we are to gain the value and the joy in life that the Giver of life would hand us on this side of the tunnel, we must begin to seek it and accept it day by day, one day at a time.

FIVE

Choose to Help Shape Your Future

My son, Bowen, was ten years old and playing his first year of Little League baseball with a highly competitive team. Jack, the coach, had recruited Bowen for his throwing arm; and Bowen could indeed throw the ball hard; but he had a problem with control. Halfway through the season, on the way to a state championship, Jack started Bowen at pitcher. Bowen's pitching was so terrible that day that Jack took him off the mound with the bases loaded and stuck him in right field where Bowen's spirits dropped lower than his shoelaces. When things weren't going so well in the fourth inning, the coach tried Bowen again at pitcher, but after two runs scored he threw his hat down and sent Bowen crying to the bench. As the game continued, Jack overcame his anger at Bowen's failures and sent him outside the fence to throw some practice pitches with the assistant coach. Then, in the last inning, with the game already lost, Jack called for Bowen to return to the mound. The bases were loaded and one man was out. I was so upset with Jack for putting my son through such humiliation that I couldn't sit down. I gripped the fence, my teeth clenched, then watched in amazement as Bowen struck out the last two batters. Our team lost the game, but Bowen came through a winner. Though he had stood broken and hopeless in right field in the first inning, Bowen finished the game as a better young man. A terrible experience in the first inning became a tolerable experience after the success in the last inning. And there was great value within the struggle for Bowen.

Most of the difficult experiences that face us with a doctor's bad news loom somewhere in the future. You might see your own future as some cloud formation that reminds you of a terrible creature just out of reach. You may feel like my son did in the beginning of the ninth inning, that his future was already determined by past events without any realistic hope that he could change it. Not so. Though life may have placed a scar on the marble of your life, God is still the Master Sculptor and offers you a chisel to help complete his work.

At a recent national oncology meeting, Edwin Cassem, physician, psychiatrist, and priest, offered six goals for patients who are faced with serious illnesses such as cancer:

> How do I learn to live ill, disabled, disfigured?
> Who am I now? How can I matter?
> Do I have a new mission?
> Can this type of life be my finest hour?
> What gifts can I give?
> How do I best prepare my loved ones to live without me? (Or with my illness.)[1]

Perhaps these questions have already occurred to you since your present diagnosis. If not, then someday they should be both asked and answered. By doing so, you can help determine your future in spite of your illness or injury.

Face the Future with Hope

Hearing bad news from your doctor is like being sent from the pitcher's mound to right field in the first inning. Hopes are dashed, and the joy of the game is over. I just told you how my son had a terrible first inning experience and then changed the game into one of value by the ninth. How do we do the same when we are broken by bad news from our doctor? *We do it by responding with hope.* And just as your hopes were dashed with the doctor's bad news, your hopes can be renewed by changes that will come. I recently began asking my cancer patients who were a year or more into their diagnosis how they had felt when they first received their bad news and how their feelings had changed with time. They taught me something about the ability humans possess to transform brokenness into value over time.

1. Charles and his wife reminded me that when they were told his diagnosis, they then heard thirty minutes of thorough discussion regarding treatment and prognosis with their heads in a fog. The next morning his wife had told me, "We didn't hear anything you told us last night after you said 'leukemia.'" I then repeated my entire discussion, and this second time they understood. *If your diagnosis brings a mental fog, you can find clarity.*
2. Inez was diagnosed with lung cancer two years ago. "I was paralyzed by fear and felt I would die within six months. When you told me you could treat me and my friends began praying, I lost my fear." *If your diagnosis brings fear, someday there can be courage.*
3. Patty's breast cancer returned in her abdomen. "I was always in charge. My hardest thing was to quit being superwoman. I guess I'll just have to be human." *If your diagnosis breaks you down, it may allow you to find your true humanity.*
4. Keith was only thirty-eight years old and diagnosed with acute leukemia. "I thought of my children at home. I knew that things were going to change, but I would do what I had to do for my kids." *If your diagnosis brings deep concern for your loved ones, that concern can be transformed into determination.*
5. Linda said when learning of her colon cancer, "My mind was blown; I was afraid of dying. I acted like I

wasn't because I didn't want my mother to worry. She was afraid too, but she acted like it was okay because she didn't want me to worry. Now we can talk about it." *If your diagnosis brings isolation, someday there can be openness.*

6. Dorothy had a cancer of her skin. "I was afraid it was going to spread all over my body and take my life. Then I came to your office and saw so many people worse off than me that I began to feel better about my situation." *If you fear the worst, someday you can find perspective.*
7. Tracey felt a knot on her neck. Her mother had died two years earlier from a cancer that began as a knot on her neck. "I felt that everything my mother went through was about to happen to me." Tracey is now cured of her lymphoma. *If your fears link you to another's fate, someday you will find your own destiny.*
8. Jean was sixty-five years old and had been diagnosed with bone lymphoma four and a half years earlier. "I was totally dazed at first without any worthwhile thoughts, but I was later able to turn it over to God. After that I had no fear, no anxiety." *If your diagnosis brings chaos, someday there can be peace.*

These are just a few examples of how patients react when they first receive bad news from their doctor and how, over time, they convert that initial tragic news into something of value. No patient I surveyed told me, "It was so terrible that I couldn't handle it, and then it became worse than I had feared." God has built into all of us the incredible ability to take a bad situation and with time bring value out of it. It is the same with any diagnosis, whether it be cancer or diabetes. Every terrible diagnosis carries within it the hope that life with value will follow. So, what can you do at the time you first receive the bad news to begin the process toward value in the future?

Every terrible diagnosis carries within it the hope that life with value will follow.

What can you do to direct your future rather than let your future direct you?

FACE THE FUTURE WITH UNDERSTANDING

In order to act effectively toward a better future, we must first understand what the future holds. Bad news from the doctor always comes to us with a sense of shock and disorientation. We often see ahead of us only the shape of a dark dragon in the shadows of the forest—terrible but undefined. When our initial mental haze clears, in order to fight the dragon we must clearly define its eyes, ears, teeth, and tail. When the fuzziness of shock wears off, you need to schedule an appointment to return to your doctor and begin to discover the details of the beast that confronts you.

Your future after the bad news will be changed. You need to learn from the doctor three things in order to begin the process of shaping your new future:

1. How will this diagnosis affect the length of my life?
2. How will this diagnosis affect the quality of my life?
3. How will the treatment affect both?

Obtaining the best treatment possible, as we discussed in a previous chapter, is vital. But so is the issue of quality of life. The quality of any person's life is the sum of all the things that make living worthwhile. How will the diagnosis and treatment alter those things that bring value to your life? What changes must you anticipate in order to continue to find value in your life in face of this bad news you have received? Soon after you receive your difficult diagnosis, I recommend you sit down with your doctor to ask him or her specifically these quality-of-life questions:

1. What physical symptoms should I anticipate as a result of my diagnosis or treatment? Will there be pain? Will there be physical disability? Should I anticipate gastrointestinal, urinary, sexual, or neurological symptoms? Physical symptoms vary tremendously from patient to patient, even among those with the same disease. Some folks with heart problems still play tennis, while others are confined to slow walks. Some with lupus have no symptoms, while others run high fevers and have strokes. Every person is different in some ways from others with their diagnosis and the same in other ways. In order to plan your future, you must, as clearly as you can determine, anticipate physical changes that will come into your life.

2. What psychological changes should I anticipate? Will the medicine make me hyperactive? Am I at risk for depression? Many women do very well emotionally as they take chemotherapy after breast cancer surgery but then slip into a depression when treatment is over. If you can anticipate psychological factors that accompany your diagnosis or treatment, you will be better prepared to prevent or deal with them.

3. What social changes will come into my life with this bad news? Will this illness I am facing make me a burden to my family, or will the difficulties of my diagnosis bring my family closer together? If I can have no children, should I adopt? Can my spouse bear the weight of my illness? Will I need help with transportation? Will I need help at home? Can I still play bridge with my friends on Wednesdays? Must I stay away from church in case there are sick people there who will give me their colds? Can I continue to work where my friends are? Will people accept me? Much of the value in our lives comes from our relationships with those with whom we spend time. You need to know whether all of that will change so you can take the steps necessary to continue to find value in relationships.

4. What is all this going to cost me? How well will my insurance take care of this? Are there options to therapy that cost different amounts? What is the economic impact of this diagnosis? Will I lose my job? You must pursue these questions in case you need to change your expenditures and lifestyle to adapt to the financial changes this bad news brings.

5. What pleasure in my life will disappear because of this bad news? One patient never focused on the life-threatening danger of his lung cancer because his greatest concern was how he could get back to playing golf. Pleasures bring us joy. These pleasures often disappear or become altered in some way because of our diagnosis. You need to ask your doctor: Will I play golf again? Can I go fishing? Will I be able to see well enough to read? Can I enjoy sex with my spouse again? How do I water ski with one leg? Pleasures are important; they must not disappear from your life when bad news comes. If the old pleasures must vanish, seek new ones to replace them.

6. Will I be able to accomplish my goals for life anymore? Achievement is critical to life satisfaction. A motivational speaker once asked his audience: "How do you know if you have had a good day?" His answer: "You've had a good day when you've made progress toward a worthwhile goal." Human beings have within them the desire to accomplish goals. When bad news from the doctor brings changes to your life, it is a good time to reassess your goals. Some of those goals may never have been possible; others have now been made impossible by your new diagnosis. What do you really want to achieve now? To find value in life, you need to set goals and pursue them. These goals must be realistic, based on the facts of your new physical state. Don't mourn old goals that have to be set aside. Instead, make new ones and pursue them each day. Remember, you've had a good day when you've made progress toward a worthwhile goal.

After you have asked the doctor these six questions regarding expected life changes, there are two more questions, critical life questions, that you should ask yourself.

7. Should I choose length of life or quality of life? Some people, when struck by tragic illness, are confronted with this most difficult of questions. Amost always, the answer I would give is, "Both!" There is something in our culture that assumes you have to choose one or the other. But even with cancer patients, most often the treatment that promises my patients the longest life also promises the best quality of life. Of course, this is not always true. I would recommend you clarify with your doctor the following:

a. How long am I likely to live without the treatment? (shortest, longest, average)
b. How long am I likely to live with the treatment? (shortest, longest, average)
c. What will my life be like without the treatment? (best, worst, average)
d. What will my life be like with the treatment? (best, worst, average)

Take these facts, discuss them with your family, pray about them, and make your best decision. Remember one important concept as you do so: quality of life is not only the quantity of pleasure and pain in your life; quality of life comes also in the good we contribute to the lives of others. God did not place us here for ourselves alone, and sometimes we gain life's greatest quality when we continue in pain in order to provide goodness to those around us. That goodness may be a smile, a conversation of peace and encouragement, a helping hand to a fellow struggler who might not take the hand of a comfortable man, a sacrificial gift, a testimony of God's goodness in the midst of our suffering. When your own life has run out of pleasure, do not conclude that your quality of life has vanished until you have looked around to see if you can bring goodness to someone else.

8. Where do I find myself spiritually with this new understanding of my health? Do I have the relationship with God that I need to strengthen me through all that lies ahead? Do I have a spiritual community to stand by me with prayer and emotional support and physical assistance during my future difficulties? If not, perhaps it is time for you to return to your spiritual roots or seek God in a way you may never have known. More than one of my patients has said, "This illness brought me back to God, and it was worth it."

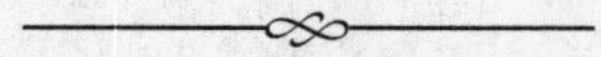

When the doctor gives you bad news, this array of questions you face and need to answer may seem overwhelming. But I do not lay them out to overwhelm or frighten you. These questions are tools that you should take to the doctor and to your family. You should use them to remodel your future as one remodels a house. You must take each of these questions and pair them up with the following four statements to lay a foundation for a new and worthwhile future:

> I will not lose; I will substitute.
>
> I will not stop; I will turn.
>
> I am here for others, not just myself.
>
> I am not alone; God and those I love are with me.

When the doctor gives you bad news and you are forced to face a different future, that future is one you have a big part in shaping. Even with a broken body, you can refuse to accept a broken life as your destiny.

TAX DEDUCTIBLE ITEM ➡ ☐

DO NOT USE
FOR REORDERING

6592

✔ Track Your Expenses…

☐ Mortgage / Rent ☐ Transportation ☐ Entertainment & Travel
☐ Gas / Electric ☐ Credit Card ☐ Medical / Dental
☐ Telephone ☐ Taxes ☐ Dependent Care
☐ Food ☐ Insurance (Life, Home, Auto) ☐ Savings & Investment
☐ Clothing ☐ Home Improvement (Maintenance, Repairs) ☐ Other ________

Nov. 17, 2005

New York & Presb Hospital

Thirty two dollars and 66/100

BAL. FOR'D	
THIS PAYMENT	32.66
BALANCE	
OTHER	
BAL. FOR'D	

…Here's How:

- Carry balance forward
- Check type of expense
- Add details on memo line
- Retain duplicates in Deluxe Check box

Memo 0510183822

⑆296075810⑆ 8100542474⑈ 06592

NOT NEGOTIABLE

WD-DUP (3)

SIX

Run to the God You Can Trust

Believing that God is involved in healing requires an intellectual choice. Knowing that God is there requires trust. For some reason God chooses to be most apparent in our lives when we most trust him. What is this thing called trust? How do we grab hold of it when the floor of our life is caving in?

Katelyn was twelve when she was diagnosed with acute leukemia. In the midst of her treatment, she developed a severe brain infection that led to a coma. Within that coma, Katelyn suffered violent seizures, underwent multiple brain operations, and was given no real hope for recovery. Katelyn's parents and God's people prayed anyway. Thousands of prayers were lifted up for Katelyn over her thousand-day illness.

Just prior to the start of Katelyn's seizures, a woman had met with Katelyn's mother and handed her a blanket that had been prayed over by a hundred nurses.

"This is for your little girl," the woman said. "She's going to get worse before she gets better, but that child is going to be fine."

A few weeks later, after the terrible seizures had begun, Katelyn was sent home on Christmas Eve to die. But Katelyn didn't die, and no one quit praying through month after month of coma; and through those prayers, God was at work. As reported in our local newspaper on the Sunday after Thanksgiving, "Kate spent her thirteenth and fourteenth birthdays breathing and eating through tubes. Last Tuesday, she spent her fifteenth birthday breathing and eating and laughing on her own, wheeling herself around her home. Her Mom and Dad and big sister spent the day being thankful."[1]

God stepped down the stairway of prayer and with his power turned the impossible into the possible for a broken little girl. What about you? Can you reach for a God who will use his power for you now, in your situation?

DOES HIS HAND REALLY REACH DOWN THIS FAR?

His shop was built like so many other buildings in Sanubi, Nigeria—stick frame packed with mud, covered by a tin roof. He probably was thirty-five, but the years had been hard for him, making him appear older. I don't know how a Nigerian blacksmith learned to speak English so well, but he did, and he welcomed me into his shop. His anvil was typical of those I have seen in western movies but different in that it was covered with the blood of a recently slaughtered chicken. On the wall was a reed mat with feathers signifying his *juju*.

"Can you tell me about the blood and the sacrifice?" I asked.

"The iron god makes my work good and protects my tools from thieves."

We talked about his understanding of his gods. Along with the iron god, he believed there were many other gods in the world that could be approached with the appropriate sacrifice to do his bidding. The blacksmith also believed in a creator god. The creator god was somehow manifested in all of creation, vaguely linked to the smaller, useful gods in the world, but the creator god was indifferent and distant in his attitude toward humankind and could not be counted on to become involved in our affairs. After I left the blacksmith, I realized that his approach to his gods was much like many Americans' approach to their God.

Throughout the world there are all kinds of ideas about who God is, what God is like, and whether God wishes to be involved in our affairs. Many people agree with the Sanubi blacksmith. They believe God exists but that he is distant and would rarely wish to become embroiled in the human condition. Some believe God may be there, just as the stars are there, but that he does not impact their life in any real way. Others believe that God may care, but he has little power to accomplish meaningful changes in individual situations.

Perhaps you have ignored the question of God's power altogether but now are reaching for any hand that might pull you out of a terrible illness or injury. If there is a God who cares and who has the power to intervene in your life for your benefit, you may wish that you had found him while you were healthy, but it is even more critical that you find him now as you face serious health problems. One thing is certain: we are inadequate, in our own power, to make life turn out the way we wish.

Recently I heard a story of a young father who was deer hunting with his best friend. His friend aimed to shoot a deer behind the shoulder blade. He could feel the excitement as he waited for the deer to drop. But it was the young father who was struck by the bullet, and all the power from human anguish in the world could not bring him back to life.

The other day I realized my own powerlessness in life. I was driving home from work and pulled into the driveway, oblivious to my immediate surroundings. My son, Bowen, had heard me coming and ran into the driveway. One second earlier and he would have been crushed by my own car, with my hands on the steering wheel.

We are powerless to control that which matters most. We demand a source of power in this world beyond ourselves to face both health and sickness. Can and will God provide for us the power we need?

While I was working in Albania this past year, faced with an impossible responsibility in both health care and in witness, I came across a verse that took hold of me and captured my attention in such a way that I read it daily for weeks. "His divine power has given us everything we need for life and godliness through our knowledge of him who called us by his own glory and goodness" (2 Peter 1:3). His divine power has given us everything we need for life. All the power we need. Everything.

How much power does it take to hold a young son with acute leukemia? Tom and Margaret know. They watched their son Eric suffer through debilitating chemotherapy to treat his childhood leukemia and waited five years until they were certain he was cured.

How much power does it take to face unemployment in middle age with no prospects? Bob, Bernie, Jerry, and Roger know. All are friends of mine who faced life in their forties and fifties looking for work.

How much power does it take to sit at your mother's bedside and push morphine until the pain goes away? My wife, Becky, knows. She sat beside her mother and held back her suffering with morphine until Nana let go of this life in exchange for heaven.

How much power do we need for life? Tom, Margaret, Bob, Bernie, Jerry, Roger, Becky, and I would say, "More than I have." But each of us would also say, "God's power was sufficient to bring me through." The apostle Peter, in that verse, is saying, "Whatever it takes for life, his power is enough."

But can God really do the big things? And will he use his power for me?

A young minister who loved the Lord died recently of his cancer. He should have died six years before, after his disease had recurred twice in his brain and in his eyes. At that time we had exhausted all measures for therapy, and I told him that he would likely die soon. This past year, five years from my pronouncement, he sat in good health in my exam room and said, "When you told me that nothing more could be done, Doc, I changed my prayer. I had been praying, 'God help me get through all of these treatments.' When you told me you had run out of stuff to do, I changed my prayer to 'God of creation, my creator and king, Master of the entire universe, please make these spots go away.' On the next MRI, you remember, Doc, no one could find my cancer."

Eventually this man's cancer took him to heaven, but it did so in God's timing, six years later than I had assumed, with God's understanding of this man's mission in life, and God's knowledge of his family's needs. God's power is real, and he uses it for real people like this minister, and you and me.

But how does God decide when to use his power? Whatever God's actions are toward us, they are motivated by goodness. God's very nature is goodness. God wishes blessings for our lives, not suffering. Any law he gives us is for our benefit. Any suffering that comes into our lives either comes to us from Satan, or it comes from a God of love. If it comes from our God of love, he is either tugging on our bridle to keep us from turning down a dangerous path or accomplishing through us a purpose that is greater than our pain, just as he did with his own Son on the Cross.

Last week I stood at the bedside of a young man dying of a brain tumor. His wife loved him dearly, and he had small children at home. When I turned away from the tragedy of that life lost too soon, I saw a note written by his family in magic marker on the board at the foot of his bed, "God is good all the time."

Another patient, Frank, was only fifty-five, and his abdomen was filled with colon cancer. We had tried our best to control the cancer but knew we would not succeed. His daughter had flown in from out of town and was standing at his bedside with her hand on his shoulder. "Daddy, before this sickness you didn't know God. But now you know him, and you will live forever." In tears and with great love for her father, she added, "That makes this worth it."

These families had found the goodness of God within the suffering of those they loved.

Whatever happens, whatever is causing your pain, God has either brought it to you in love or will step in where Satan has trod and make good grow out of evil (Rom. 8:28).

Pray this simple prayer: *Dear God, your divine power has given me everything I need for life, for godliness, and for this situation. Let me reach for your hand that I may feel your goodness and see it work in my life now. Amen.*

HOW DO I FIND THE STRENTH TO REACH FOR HIS HAND?

Sometimes we know that God is there (with all of our hearts) but just don't have the strength to reach for him. Let me give you three steps you can take to find God's hand when your faith is real but your heart is weak.

LOOK BACKWARD

Tyler Henry was riding my son's four-wheeler deep in the woods when it struck a tree, flipped over, and cut his leg wide open. My son had to run through the forest to civilization and find help to bring

Tyler out of the woods. I saw the wound in disbelief. The back of the leg was sliced open from the knee to the ankle, all the way to the bone, with muscle flapping freely as our car rushed toward the emergency room. The wound was filled with leaves and dirt. For many reasons, Tyler's wound was not cleaned and repaired for more than twelve hours. His chance for a major infection was over 90 percent. His chance of losing the leg was great. People prayed. God touched that wound of more than a thousand stitches and healed it without the slightest complication. As I look back on that young man and his parents who trusted the Father, the trust they had in God has become one of my present pillars of faith.

I'm not the first to look back and find faith. The Israelites had wandered in the desert for forty years because of their failure to trust God. Then they came to face the Jordan, like an arrow in the bow of God, to be propelled into the Promised Land. Rather than rousing them with the promise and excitement of events ahead, Moses had them look back over the past forty years (Deut. 1–3). Why did he do that? I thought *faith* meant we trusted God to do something for us in the future.

Have you ever held up a bow with an arrow notched in the string, pointed in the right direction, and then asked the arrow to move forward and strike the target? It doesn't work. The arrow simply sits there. In spite of all your verbal appeals to convince the arrow to charge ahead, and regardless of the beauty of the target, the arrow will not move forward until something happens. What is that something? The string must be pulled *back* to provide the power necessary to propel the arrow *forward* to its destination.

Sometimes we think faith is simply looking forward and believing something will happen. But much of the power of faith comes from looking back on what God has already done in our lives and trusting that he can do it again. You may now be in trouble with your health. What has God done in your life before this crisis that will enable you to trust him with your situation now? When I face crises in my own life, I look back and realize that what God did for Israel he has also done for me. As Moses spoke to the children of Israel regarding God's past actions in their lives, he was also speaking to me.

He created me. "Ask now about the former days, long before your time, from the day God created man on the earth; ask from one end of the heavens to the other. Has anything so great as this ever happened, or has anything like it ever been heard of?" (Deut. 4:32).

He has spoken to me. "Has any other people heard the voice of God speaking out of fire, as you have, and lived?" (Deut. 4:33).

He has acted in my life. "Has any god ever tried to take for himself one nation out of another nation, by testings, by miraculous signs and wonders, by war, by a mighty hand and an outstretched arm, or by great and awesome deeds, like all the things the Lord your God did for you in Egypt before your very eyes?" (Deut. 4:34).

He has been with me. "Because he loved your forefathers and chose their descendants after them, he brought you out of Egypt by his Presence and his great strength" (Deut. 4:37).

Faith comes from looking back: looking back on his Word, looking back on his actions in your life, looking back on the times his presence was real in your life. God has held me, and he will hold me again. He has shown me the way, and he will show me again. His Word has been real and true in my life, so I can seek guidance and truth from him now.

I periodically travel to Albania to work with Albanian doctors in developing their health-care system. On a recent trip, a young Albanian pastor explained in a different way his understanding of faith. Faith, he said, is moving through life as if we were rowing a boat toward our destination. As we row, our backs are actually facing our destination, and we are watching for direction from our Pilot, who can see clearly from his position standing in the rear of the boat. As he tells us to pull harder on the right oar or harder on the left, we continue to move in the direction he chooses, not knowing what our Pilot sees. Then, as we see our life moving past us, we realize his direction was true, and we gain confidence that he will take us where we wish to be.

Many of my cancer patients are so shocked by the flashing storm ahead that for a time they fail to remember what God has done for them in the past. Now, as you face an uncertain and difficult future with your health, make the choice: look back over your life and see the footprints of God and know that he will carry you through this trial as well.

Deal with Uncertainty

Total trust—our eyes on the Pilot, remembering his faithfulness, confident of the future—this is the ideal for our lives. But what if we're not quite there yet? What if we still feel the anxiety of uncertainty ahead?

Sandy was young; she had a lot of life ahead of her. She also had breast cancer. Five lymph nodes under her arm demonstrated evidence of disease, which gave her a 50 percent chance of dying from breast cancer. To improve her chances of survival, we chose to treat her with aggressive chemotherapy. Breast cancer is a disease that must be stopped before it appears in the lungs, bone, liver, or brain. After it has spread to these organs, it can rarely be cured. Sandy understood this, and we pushed ahead. She took the harsh treatments like a champion.

After the first three rounds of therapy, Sandy was without hair but otherwise was holding up well physically. We performed bone and liver scans to be certain we were still without evidence of spread before moving to the next phase of treatment. Unlike her initial scans, there now were subtle changes in her bones and liver. Our radiologist is a pessimist and called them cancer. I'm an optimist and believed these changes were too nonspecific to definitely be called cancer. The uncertainty nearly destroyed Sandy. If cancer was not there, her chances for cure were good. But if the spots on the scans were cancer, it would kill her. There were no reasonable tests to end the uncertainty. The truth is, I *thought* Sandy would be all right, but I couldn't give her the absolute certainty she needed. At this point it was not her cancer but the uncertainty that was so devastating to Sandy.

When we ponder our own serious health problems, it is the uncertainty surrounding our illness that is often so difficult. Well-meaning people who are not facing our trial themselves will tell us, "I think you will be all right," or even, "You are going to be all right." But we know that most don't know; they have never been there. They are talking about hope, not certainty. Uncertainty often causes suffering. But uncertainty is a door that can swing both ways—into times of great sorrow or into times of great joy.

I don't have a very good memory, but one of the few solid memories of my childhood is that of Christmas morning. When I was young we lived in a two-story house with a winding stairway in the entrance hall. After we four children awakened our parents on Christmas morning, we were required to wait at the top of the stairs while my father put together his movie camera and lights. The lights were a monstrosity—four large floodlights attached to a four-foot bar connected to a handle on which the camera was mounted. When this equipment was finally assembled, we were allowed to descend the stairs, one at a time, staring into those blinding lights, waving on cue. To us, all the important stuff was beyond those lights, in the living room under the Christmas tree. We could never be certain, as we stood at the top of the stairs waiting our turn, that what we would find under the tree was what we had asked for and dreamed of. In spite of that, we were excited and confident rather than fearful and anxious. We were confident that Christmas morning would bring us joy because we knew the man who had prepared that morning for us. We had lived with him and seen him in action. We knew his character. We knew his love for us. And we had never been disappointed. We remembered from Christmases past that we did not always find what we expected under the tree, but whatever we received was always wonderful. As I revisit those memories, I find it interesting that I do not remember any of the gifts I received, but I remember with great joy and great love my father hidden by the floodlights, waiting for us at the bottom of the stairs.

The way to change an uncertainty that fears the worst to an uncertainty that expects the best is to know the one at the bottom of the stairs.

Uncertainty is uncertainty, whether it surrounds a Christmas morning or an experience with serious illness. The difference is that with sickness or impending death, uncertainty imagines the worst rather than the best. The way to change an uncertainty that fears the worst to an uncertainty that expects the best is to know the one at the bottom of the stairs.

Jesus said it this way, "Which of you, if his son asks for bread, will give him a stone? Or if he asks for a fish, will give him a snake? If you, then, though you are evil, know how to give good gifts to your children, how much more will your Father in heaven give good gifts to those who ask him!" (Matt. 7:9–11).

A breast cancer patient sent me a birthday card with the same message:

> I said to the man who stood at the gate of the years,
> "Give me light, that I may tread safely into the unknown."
> And he replied:
> "Go out into the darkness and put your hand into the hand of God.
> That shall be to you better than light and safer than the known way."[2]

Let us get to know the Father who awaits us. When we truly know him, we can trust him. When we trust him, we can expect the best because we know the one at the bottom of the stairs.

Walk in Obedience

Trust comes from looking back. Trust comes when we make uncertainty our friend and expect the best. Trust comes most solidly when we walk ahead with God in obedience, whatever the fears and consequences.

I have found this to be true in my own life. I've been a Christian since my youth and have loved and trusted God since that time, but it was years before I overcame my fear of death. In spite of my Christian faith, there were nights I would lie awake contemplating the end of life with cold sweats and great fear. When I turned thirty-three, my life underwent a major change. Becky and I had been clearly called to foreign missions and were headed in that direction—leaving my private practice, selling our home—when Becky became pregnant with our second child. Becky became deathly ill, at first physically ill with nausea, vomiting, weight loss, and weakness. I had to carry her in my arms to the bathroom. Then she became severely depressed. We came to the point, in spite of all the medical help available, that I honestly thought she might die from either her physical or psychological illness. I had prayed and cried for weeks, but God never spoke. Here we were, following God's call to missions with all our hearts and actions, and we were broken, with no hope.

We entered the hospital for an abortion. We knew it was against our faith. We knew it would end our hope of foreign missions. We knew that a baby would die. And in despair, we planned to proceed. Prior to the abortion, my father walked into Becky's hospital room and said, "I love you more than anything in the world. I know that what I'm going to tell you may make you turn away from me forever. But what you are planning to do is wrong." He then walked out of the room, and Becky and I poured out our remaining tears, holding each other in our arms.

When we had finished crying, we committed to God that we would go through the pregnancy regardless of the outcome. Almost immediately Becky was better. Her sickness became manageable. She began gaining weight and strength. Six months later, Catherine was born. When she was six weeks old, we took her with us to Nigeria. What I remember most in looking back on that experience are two things: The first was the feeling of falling hopelessly and desperately, then landing in the arms of God. The second was the realization that from that experience until now, I have rarely again felt the fear of death.

I learned a number of truths within that experience that impact my life as I look toward my future. I realized first that God wants our obedience even when we don't feel like giving it. Even when there is no peace or joy in walking with him, he still expects us to walk with him and obey. We are not creatures who must follow our emotions. We are creatures who must carry our emotions with us as we follow God. Then, as we become liberated from the demands of our feelings, we discover that our sack of joy and peace eventually overflows beyond its previous capacity. "Delight yourself in the LORD and he will give you the desires of your heart" (Ps. 37:4).

Second, I discovered that when we obey, we are allowed to see God. Deitrich Bonhoeffer said, "Only he who sees, obeys; but only he who obeys, sees."[3] It has always been the case in my life that God has revealed himself most clearly when I was following him in obedience.

Before I committed to obey God's will for our child, I was afraid of death, and I had never fully realized what it felt like to fall into the arms of God. But then, by obeying against my desire, in spite of my emotions, I experienced God in a way not possible otherwise. And somehow by feeling God's arms around me, my fear of death was taken away. I did not rationalize, "God is great, therefore I should not fear death." I simply experienced God and realized my fear was gone.

I also learned again that God works through his people. If left on our own with the best medical science and our best energies, we would have aborted Catherine. She would never have grown up to dream of Olympic gymnastics or sleep on our floor and say in the dark, "Good-night, I love you." But we were not on our own. God worked through my father to speak his word with intense love, and we were changed. God has chosen throughout history to work his will through the people around us. As we face each of life's tragedies and death itself, we must open ourselves to the presence and help of God that comes through his people to us; even when we think we can make it better alone—Satan's lie.

I discovered that when we obey, we are allowed to see God.

Finally, I came to understand the arms of God. I found they were strong; they were loving; they cared even for me. It was in those arms that the fear of death dissolved. If I had never despaired, never reached the end of my possibilities, never lay trapped with no exit, I would never have felt those arms. My faith is built not only on what I read in his Word and hear from his people but also on those arms that lifted me up so well against all odds. The pain and despair of the moment was nothing compared to the joy of knowing those arms. I can look back on that terrible experience today and say, "It was worth it." And I can look forward, even as far as death, and know that those same arms are waiting to catch me there. This life-changing confidence came only because we were obedient to God in the midst of our despair.

What would God have you do in the midst of your own despair? As you struggle with all of your strength through your illness or injury, what step is God asking you to take for him? Is there a relationship he is asking you to mend? Is he asking you to let go of some special sin? Is there a mission he has asked you to complete, though you are too weary to take another step? God has not removed his purpose from your life simply because you are wounded. If you step forward to his call, particularly now when you are suffering, he will hand you a blessing that otherwise would be impossible for you to receive.

Why So Often Do We Fail to Choose Him?

As I have pondered why some whom I have known have failed to reach for God in their crises, there come to mind many individual responses. Often I find it to be a problem of focus. People in pain often focus inwardly with two distinct statements, each one a shade on the windows to their hearts, keeping out the light of God.

I Think I Can Make It on My Own

My college roommate, Phillip, and I had worked out a deal for our short spring semester. We were to get full credits in English and photography for a trip to the Washington Cascades. We would read Emerson and Thoreau, take photographs, develop them in mountain streams, keep a diary, write a book, and get full semester credit for camping out in the mountains! After the usual breakdowns, long nights on the road, and beef burgundy at my Aunt Marthel's, we parked our station wagon at the ferry lot and climbed aboard the open ferry for the ride up the fingerlike Lake Chelan to Stehekin. As we moved away from the sun, it played in our wake with its rays bouncing from one ripple to the next. Each minute sent another mountain into shades of blue as a higher more rugged one moved in to fill the vacant green.

We met Sam on the boat. He and his wife had lived in a tent for two years while they built their ranch home in the narrow Stehekin Valley years earlier. Together they had packed in five tons of granite from the mountains to build their fireplace. Now she was down the lake in a nursing home with multiple sclerosis while he remained at the ranch alone. We met him on the boat and became friends, and he offered to let us camp on his land at the foot of the mountains. I asked him if he ever became lonely with so few people around.

"Nature takes care of that problem," he said. "You don't get lonely when you spend your life in such beautiful country."

We spent a number of days talking with Sam, exploring the mountains, reading, writing, and building fences for our keep. Soon, however, Sam got tired of us and we of him. It was time to leave, but we had sworn that before we left we would climb a certain mountain that rose up fifty-six hundred feet from our valley. Phillip described our adventure in his diary:

> Today it was a mountain we had to climb. We began at 8:45 and climbed steadily for almost an hour until we came to our first big cliff. The climb up the cliff was difficult because of the loose rocks, which we watched go crashing down the mountainside. At one point I had to take my pack off to climb up a slippery ledge. Hugging the cliff with my fingernails, I began to feel myself fall, and for the first time I thought we had really pulled a good one.
>
> We were determined to reach the top, but from every slope we reached there was always another in sight. At 1:00 we finally reached our limit. Snow covered the bare rock and more snow was falling. We knew that going up those cliffs would be difficult and coming back down them would be impossible. Our descent began with hunger and more than its share of apprehension.
>
> At first we tried the water runs, but they proved to be too slippery and steeper than they looked. After two hours we had only moved a few hundred feet down and soon realized we had moved too far to the right to pick up our old trail. It wasn't just fun or adventure anymore; a man had died the year before on this mountain while trying to make it down at night.
>
> A cliff almost straight down, lined with loose rocks, was directly before us, and we nearly decided to move even further to the right. It was then that I noticed a well-worn deer path crisscrossing the slope. Deciding that if a deer could make it, we had to give it a try, we slid and squatted down the slope.

> We then came to a rock slide and the path disappeared. Just as we were thinking how lost we were, a big buck appeared on the other side of the slide and virtually flew down the mountainside. Smiling at each other, we carefully crawled across the slide and found the small hillside pasture the buck had used. We picked up his trail, and in less than an hour we were back at home."[4]

Phillip and I were young and strong and had made it up the mountain. You always figure it's going up the mountain that's tough, when in fact it is often in coming down that a person loses his way, trips, falls, and is filled with fear. So it is with life. Many struggles of building, gathering, and climbing are behind us, and we think we can handle life pretty well. Then the doctor brings us bad news. Sometimes we feel we can handle this just like we've handled everything else. If you think you can, don't let me stop you. But when you come to the edge of the cliff with no trail in sight, do not forget that God is there, willing and able to lead you down the mountain.

David knew this and called God his Shepherd. Even when things got bad enough that he knew he might die, David knew his Shepherd would lead him well. In Psalm 23 David says, "Even though I walk through the valley of the shadow of death, I will fear no evil, for you are with me" (Ps. 23:4).

Death will certainly come to each of us some day. Death may be your greatest fear now with this bad news from your doctor. God does not always protect us from death, but there is a difference in facing death with the Shepherd and facing it alone. With the Shepherd, the evil of death is gone. Our Shepherd leads us through the gate of death into eternal life. Death of a loved one may hurt more than our own, but with the Shepherd, its evil is gone also. The separation caused by death is temporary. With the Shepherd, we can look forward to a joyous reunion in eternity. Your trouble may not be an impending death but an impossible life with your health problem. It is only impossible if you face it on your own. Whether through a difficult time of life or through the gates of death, you need not walk alone; your Shepherd is there to lead you if you will choose to let him do so.

I Must Have Done Something Wrong

Sometimes we fail to reach for God's power because we misunderstand the depth of his love for us. So many people, when they face a health tragedy, whether they say it out loud or only think it, feel that they must have done something wrong in their lives and now God is getting even. If we have a past that haunts us when medical problems come to break our dreams, we can either curse God as a distant accuser, or we can turn to him as a loving father. I recently heard a story that illustrates my understanding of the Father.

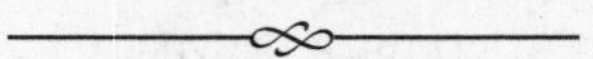

Bernie was raised by a single mother with a small income. He was quite nearsighted as a boy, but his mother had been able to buy him a pair of glasses. They were a precious instrument for him, and when the earpiece screw was lost, he kept them working with a safety pin in the hinge. Bernie's mother warned him to be careful with his glasses when he was playing, because she could not afford another pair.

One winter day at Gragg Elementary, the snow began to fall. When a couple of inches had collected on the ground, Bernie's teacher gave the class a recess to allow the students to run outside and play in the snow, for snow was a rare event in Memphis. Bernie was a responsible young boy, so he dutifully took off his glasses and placed them in his shirt pocket before putting on his coat to join the fun. After running and sliding and fighting with snowballs for a while, the teacher called them back inside to resume class.

When Bernie removed his coat, he reached for his glasses and discovered they were gone. Despair struck him. He told his teacher, who, filled with understanding, asked all the boys in the class to dress up again and go out to find the glasses. Twenty boys combed the two-acre playground as the snow continued to fall around them. No glasses.

Bernie went home, brokenhearted and afraid, and told his mother the story. She did not cry out in anger but put on her coat and walked with Bernie the cold mile and a half back to school. When they reached the schoolyard, his mother stopped and faced the field where they had been playing. The snow continued to fall, the afternoon sun was fading, and she asked her son, "Where were you when you lost them?" Bernie, frustrated, waved his hand over the entire field and said, "We went everywhere!" After a pause and a prayer, Bernie watched his mother trudge across the field. She leaned over, brushed away a layer of snow, picked up his glasses, and they walked home together.

God is good like Bernie's mom—only better. The world prepares us for illness with fear, impotence, and guilt: "You have diabetes." "You're going on dialysis." "You have lung cancer." "I'm sorry, you're on your own." But, unlike the world, God says, "I am good; I'll take care of it." Bad health is not God's angry "I told you so."

We cry out, "I've lost my glasses; it's my fault. I've done everything I can do, and they are gone, and it's cold, and it's dark, and it's over." God says, "Take my hand; I will walk with you through the cold and the dark." When we reach the schoolyard, he says, "Wait here a moment." He walks across the field, reaches down, brushes away the snow, and brings us back our glasses; then we walk home together.

God says, "Take my hand; I will walk with you through the cold and the dark."

Sometimes my patients ask me why they have to face their tragic situations. I have no simple or satisfying answer. I don't know why God chose death as the door to eternity or why he allows suffering in our lives. This is not a world in which we do not lose glasses. It is, however, a world in which we have a choice. We can either give up and leave our glasses where they lie buried, or we can reach for our Creator, who will help us find them and take us home.

Dear God, I have lost my glasses. I don't know why. My health is broken and my dreams are broken. You alone have the power to heal. Work through my doctors. Work through my prayers. Work through the prayers of those who love me. Please, show your power and make me whole again. Amen.

SEVEN

Choose the Right Battle Plan

MARTIA HAS LUNG CANCER. SHE HAS NEVER SMOKED, BUT WHEN SHE arrived in my office, she not only had cancer in her lungs but also in her liver and her brain. Her war against cancer has been difficult, but her spirit has remained strong. She is right with God, solid with her husband, and wants most of all to raise her kids to be all that God created them to be.

Martia's war against cancer started with a special high-dose radiation to the brain, followed by three different kinds of chemotherapy, each producing a minor or short-term response. Finally we were forced to hold any more chemotherapy and instead treat her with radiation to her chest and brain.

On each visit her dedicated husband is there, taking notes, asking about new treatments. He is always polite, unafraid to ask tough questions or request additional information from my office. It was Martia's husband who pushed us toward an experimental cancer drug that is effective in only 10 percent of chemotherapy failures. We were able to provide the drug, and Martia's cancer responded much better than we had expected.

Through it all Martia has been solid, always ready for the next step, tough as it might be. She is taking each treatment with the confidence that we are guiding her correctly and with the will to continue when her body and emotions tell her to sit down and quit. She is *fighting for her life* and, at the same time, *living her life*—for her kids, for her husband, with her friends, and under the umbrella of God's love.

Martia is a model for others fighting through a difficult illness. In this brief chapter I want to list for you the steps Martia is taking in her battle against cancer. You can apply these steps to your health problem, whatever it is. Most are expanded elsewhere in the book, but it helps to see the battle plan all in one place so you can use these strategies in your life and check them off as you fight.

Remain educated.

1. Understand the treatment goals—know what can and can't be accomplished. This applies not only at the time of the initial diagnosis but also with the many decisions along the way. Ask often, "Doctor, what is the goal of this procedure or treatment?"
2. Understand the complications possible from the illness and from the therapy. Be ready to alert your doctor immediately if a complication arises. Delayed care of a complication could lead to a major setback. If you are aware of problems that might arise, you can contact your doctor quickly to intervene before much harm has been done.
3. Bring your questions each time you visit your doctor. Keep a notepad at home—"Questions for the Doctor." When an idea comes up, write it down. Before your visit, review the list and scratch out any unimportant questions so the doctor will focus his or her limited time with you on your most important concerns.
4. Obtain from your doctor a printed explanation of your disease and its therapy as well as two web sites that deal with your disease and therapies. Once a month check the web sites for new information. At each visit ask your doctor, "Have you come across anything new for my illness?"

Fight the battle.

1. Don't look beyond the horizon. Choose a visible goal toward which you can direct your energies. In Martia's case I tell her, "We are going to do this for two months, then reassess. Can you go that far with me?" This goal setting would be the same for rehabilitation after surgery or a stroke. Choose step-by-step, visible, reachable goals, then fight as hard as necessary to reach those goals one at a time.
2. Remember that fighting the battles involved with your illness must be an act of will, not emotion. "I will reach that goal whether or not I feel like reaching that goal." Emotions will fluctuate, but the will and action must remain steady and persistent.
3. Plan to win. Be confident that you will reach the next goal.
4. If you fail to reach a goal, remember that it was only one step that failed, one battle that was lost, not the whole war. A failure is not a time to quit but a time to try again with a different method or in a different direction.
5. Pray daily for strength in the battle.

Establish your support. Family members, friends, church members, and professionals can be an invaluable support team. Recruit them. List them so you can see the names on a piece of paper. Don't feel guilty about asking for help. If the circumstances were reversed, you would be there for them.

Continue life outside of your illness. Too much focus on the battle against the illness will injure your ability to be human, to be loved, and to be used by God. Devote all the energy necessary to achieve your health-care goal, but not more energy or time than is necessary to achieve that goal. Life outside of your illness continues—be part of it.

Think of others. Self-focus leads to self-pity, which leads to depression and bitterness. Depression and bitterness will diminish the possibility that you will actually reach your goal.

Know what needs to be done. Organize your health care in three lists.

- What do I need to do this week?
- What does my doctor need to do this week?
- What does my support team need to do this week?

Make certain these things happen, and check them off when you are confident that all those needs are being accomplished. Then spend no more time thinking of your illness. Instead, look around you, first at your family, then at your friends, then at other hurting people, and ask yourself, "What do I need to do for them?"

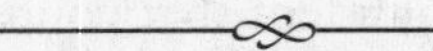

It is nearing Christmas as I write this and Martia is doing well, nine months into her illness. Each time I see Martia's name on my list of scheduled appointments, I begin to pray for her test results, and each time God has said, "Yes." God has blessed our efforts and Christmas will be fine for Martia, her husband, and her children.

Call this chapter "Martia's List." Keep it where you can review it once a week. When you follow these rules, you not only are more likely to accomplish your health-care goals, but you also are much more likely to not lose sight of what is important in your life. Sometimes it is the shock of an illness or accident that awakens us to the true value of life. And sometimes it is in the fighting of the battle for health that we come closest to realizing the true nature of God's mission for our lives.

EIGHT

Choose to Face the Tough Questions

Few of us in the Western world can imagine ground zero in Nagasaki, Japan, when the atomic bomb was dropped on August 9, 1945. Most of us identify this as the time and place our enemy was defeated, and we care to know little else. The details of that event are much more profound than we can imagine. Nagasaki was not the intended target of our military on that day with that bomb. Heavy cloud cover forced the pilot to fly there as a secondary target, important for its Mitsubishi iron works. But much of Nagasaki, including the Mitsubishi plant, was also obscured by clouds, and an alternate target within that city was chosen. The atom bomb exploded five hundred yards directly above its target, the Urakami Cathedral, centering its destruction on the neighborhood of the majority of Nagasaki's Catholic Christians. Eighty thousand people died that day.

Dr. Takashi Nagai, a Christian since 1934, walked home to find his house destroyed and his wife's charred body with her hands clutching her rosary as a last hope within the atomic storm. Rather than shaking his fist at God, Dr. Nagai told his people in an open-air requiem Mass, "We have disobeyed the law of love. Joyfully we have hated one another.... In order to restore peace to the world it was not sufficient to repent. We had to obtain God's pardon through the offering of a great sacrifice.... Let us give thanks that Nagasaki was chosen for the sacrifice."[1]

Dr. Nagai was trying to answer the *why* behind the great suffering of the Nagasaki Christians. Within that answer he found the purpose of God.

ANSWERING "WHY?" AND "WHAT HAVE I DONE?"

Dr. Nagai was attempting to answer the questions we all have when tragedy strikes: "Why?" "Why did this happen?" "What have I done?" "Why is this happening to me?" These questions I often hear from my patients.

When Jesus was asked that question, he referred to a tragedy, the collapse of a tower in Siloam that killed eighteen. "Those eighteen who died when the tower in Siloam fell on them—do you think they were more guilty than all the others living in Jerusalem? I tell you, no!" (Luke 13:4–5).

Why is it so easy to assume otherwise? Sometimes in our anguish over our suffering, we point the blame at ourselves, or at a particular person, or even at God. I heard a young woman recently recount an experience during a period of grief in her life. At the time she was a graduate student in seminary and working for her tuition as a secretary for the chairman of the New Testament division. She had lost someone she loved, and the pain would not let go. One day in her anguish, she shouted to her boss, "If another well-meaning person tells me that I should thank God because this is his will, I'm going to scream!"

The New Testament scholar looked at her in his own near anger, pointed his finger at her, and in his distinctive Nova Scotia brogue replied, "Don't you ever thank God for something that breaks his heart!" Then he dropped his finger, relaxed his face, and added, "But you can thank him that he is in this struggle with you and will see you through."

I often face this misunderstanding of God's will in my patients. One man I knew lay agitated and disoriented from the brain tumor that was sucking his life away with no further treatment possible. His wife sat on the couch beside me as we discussed the misery ahead and his eventual death.

"I'm sorry you're having to go through this," I said.

"That's okay," she answered. "We didn't plan it. God planned it."

I had heard that statement before and felt the pain of that answer, and I spoke again, hesitantly, "I don't know what God plans on this earth and what he doesn't plan. It seems that sometimes when we suffer he withholds the hand that could stop that suffering. But I know we can trust the hand. It's the same hand he withheld when his own Son was suffering for me. I know that whatever he plans grows out of his love for me."

There was a time when I was certain that God never caused the suffering of his faithful—that only sin and Satan brought suffering—but I probably was wrong.

Sometimes in our anguish, we point the blame at ourselves, or even at God.

A few weeks ago Tom, the husband of a former patient, stopped me in the hall of the West Clinic. His wife, Janice, had died five years before due to complications of the treatment I had given her for cancer. Though we had been fighting desperately to hold back an incurable cancer, the treatment had actually shortened her life. As Janice was dying, I explained to the family that the medicine I gave her had led to her death.

Now, five years later, Tom stopped me in the hall, and I was startled. I hadn't seen him since the death of his wife. He said he had been thinking a great deal about Janice lately and had planned to write me a letter.

Tom told me that he had been quite angry with me after his wife's death, and that anger had stayed with him for some time. But over the years he had come to a different understanding. He said Janice had been a special person. By that he meant more than just that she was nice; he meant she was a special person morally and spiritually. He said Janice had a connection with God that other people did not have. He told me that just before the recurrence of her cancer, their son had had his second recurrence of a different type of cancer, this time on the surface of his liver. At the time, Janice had asked quite sincerely, "Lord, take me instead of him."

Since his wife's death, Tom said he had come to the firm understanding that Janice had not died solely because she had received the toxic medicine. Instead, he said, God had answered a mother's prayer and had accepted her as a sacrifice to save their son. Tom believed I was the instrument God had used in that sacrifice, and he had come to forgive me for my part in Janice's death.

I have often felt the desire to be God's instrument to ease people's suffering so they might live. This is the first time someone has named me as an instrument used by God to bring about someone's death for a greater purpose, that of saving the life of a son. Their son is still healthy and doing fine.

The older I get, the less confident I become that I can understand the cause of anyone's suffering. I don't know how often God causes suffering in his people to bring about his purpose in this world. But I know that God's purpose is good and that it is done in love. Therefore, how great must be the purpose he is accomplishing if it requires my suffering when he loves me so much.

Lettie B. Cowman put it a different way:

> Chance has not brought this ill to me;
> It's God's own hand, so let it be,
> For He sees what I cannot see.
> There is a purpose for each pain,
> And He one day will make it plain
> That earthly loss is heavenly gain.
> Like as a piece of tapestry
> Viewed from the back appears to be
> Only threads tangled hopelessly;
> But in the front a picture fair
> Rewards the worker for his care,
> Proving his skill and patience rare.
> You are the Workman, I the frame.
> Lord, for the glory of Your Name,
> Perfect Your image on the same.[2]

Sometimes we strain to answer the question "Why?" in theological terms, with Scripture to back our interpretation. I'm not sure that God often wishes to answer the question "Why?" when we face tragedy, but I believe it is human and right to ask the question. A poignant scene in the rock musical *Jesus Christ Superstar* depicts Jesus at Gethsemane. Jesus is struggling with the path to the Cross that lay ahead, and he cries out, "Why must I die?" Then he continues to say to God, "You're awfully good at what and where but not so good at why."

That statement from the musical has been true of most suffering I have witnessed. I believe the question "Why?" that follows the tragedies of life usually is never answered in this life. Yet, even though we may never receive an answer, we can rest in the arms of the only one who holds the answer. We cannot understand, but we can trust.

I'm not sure that God often wishes to answer "Why?" but I believe it is right to ask.

Ellen McCall was able to do that. She was my best friend's mother and the National Mother of the Year the last year of her life. As she traveled the country in speaking engagements, ovarian cancer slowly drained the human life from her. In spite of the pain and the knowledge of her approaching death, she proclaimed in her speeches, "I know not what tomorrow holds, but I know who holds tomorrow." As you face your own suffering, you can diminish its torment if you will also diminish the importance of the question, "Why me?" and replace it with a growing trust in God.

A companion question to "Why me?" is the question, "Now that I'm here, where are you, God?" Sometimes God is obviously present and heals people miraculously. William had had a large melanoma removed from his thigh the year before he came to me. He was complaining of back pain, and a full evaluation revealed a mass above his kidney on the left. Needle biopsy demonstrated malignant melanoma. It was there; I saw the mass on the X-ray film. I referred him to the National Cancer Institute for experimental management. When they evaluated him, the mass was gone. God took it away.

I know firsthand that God heals miraculously. I told you how I, as an infant, did not mature as I should have. I didn't sit or communicate as I should because of a degeneration of my brain. Appropriate surgery and drainage were performed, but the neurosurgeon told my parents I would either die or become a vegetable. I did neither. My best friend used to tease me that I had fooled everyone and had become a fruit instead.

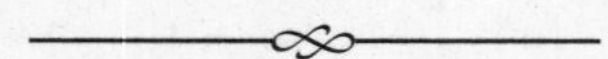

Everyone has a different definition of a miracle. I believe our definitions are too narrow and that each day we live is a miracle of God's creative and sustaining power. However we define miracle, at least some of the cases I've described, such as David and the snake bite or William and his melanoma, would fit most average people's definition. In each situation, science said there was no hope, and healing came despite that pronouncement. I believe miracles do happen. God sometimes reaches down in extraordinary ways to change the result of an illness or injury, going against the laws of science. Most of us facing death someday will pray for this kind of miracle, and most of us will be disappointed. Most of us will follow the consequences of God's natural laws and the understanding of medical science and die somewhere near the time our physician predicts.

Why don't miracles always happen?

Where is God when I am facing death and need him most?

Why doesn't he use his power to save me?

These are the tough questions. These are the questions that usually go unanswered. In twenty-five years of facing patients who ask such questions, I've learned there are no pat answers. However, there are five signposts I've used to keep me on God's trail as I travel through the forest of tough questions.

1. We do not understand the why behind most suffering (Isa. 55:8–9). It is good to ask the question, for in a few cases there is an answer. God may be using the experience like a bit in the mouth of a horse that is galloping toward a dangerous cliff. There may have been an action in my life for which this was the natural consequence. The experience may have been the only way to open the door to an opportunity for tremendous good. Or, as Joni Eareckson Tada said, "Asking 'why' is good. It establishes a relationship with the only one who has the answers."[3] It is good to ask why, but most of the time we will not hear the answer.

2. Each day of our life has been a miraculous gift; we must not lose our faith because of the exceptional days in which that miracle seems to be withheld (Ps.139:13–14). Sometimes it is the shock of an illness or accident that can awaken us to the reality of the true value of life. Frankie was only thirty-five, too young to have lung cancer. Thank God she was cured. But in the midst of her battle against that cancer, she told me, "My life is so different now than before. I get up every day just grateful that I'm alive. I don't understand how so many people can be tired and depressed each day. I've got cancer, and I spend my days helping them. I'm just excited about living each day."

3. There are no good answers unless we see life in an eternal time frame (2 Cor. 4:17–18). As hard as we may try, we cannot make sense or find justice in every event in our lives if we confine our focus to this side of eternity. If there were no life after death, most of our suffering in this world would be wasted. But there is life after death. Death is a gate to heaven, not a cliff we fall off. God will make all things right someday, sometimes soon, sometimes later.

4. The ultimate answers to all of these tough questions come in knowing God (Job 42:1–6). There is something about being face-to-face with the Father who loves us that removes the weight of terrible questions. On the same tape mentioned above, Joni Eareckson Tada told the story of a patient with Lou Gehrig's disease who was faced with the question of whether to stay alive on a ventilator. Joni said she had no clear answer, and after struggling over what to say, she found herself singing softly to the patient,

> "I must tell Jesus all of my trials
> I cannot bear my burdens alone. . . ."[4]

Sometimes the best way to relieve ourselves of the heavy burden of our questions is to lay them at the feet of the God who loves us.

5. We can trust our God to bring good even out of our disasters (Rom. 8:28). God is with us. God is good. He will bring good even out of our greatest tragedies. Our suffering is not wasted.

Jimmy was a bear of a guy with a new cancer that frightened the stuffing out of him. Two years after his diagnosis he told me, "You know, Satan messed up. He meant to drive me away from God with this cancer, but the truth is, it just drove me closer to him. It was worth all I've been through."

Sometimes we see the good our trouble brings; sometimes we don't. Sometimes we feel the loving arms of God as they carry us; sometimes we don't. But God is with us in our tragedy, and we can trust him; great good will come out of great suffering when we know him.

Sometimes it helps to look at those who have gone before us. I mentioned my best friend's mother, Ellen McCall. I remember her as being so full of life and as the only person I knew who could pronounce my name, "Al," with two syllables. I loved her as a second mother. She lived with her cancer a few years before it took her life. As she endured her suffering, knowing that she would soon die, she loudly and joyously proclaimed the love and power of God.

It is the same for Mary, a thirty-nine-year-old patient of mine with lung cancer. The cancer has spread to her bones and, as hard as I try to stop her cancer, it continues to progress very painfully. She describes her sickness and pain very objectively, but never with bitterness. Often, when I have completed my work with Mary, her parting words will be, "I love you, Dr. Weir." She recently entered the hospital with a fracture in her right leg due to the cancer. She went into surgery to have the fracture stabilized and did well during surgery, but she awakened the next morning unable to move her legs. She was paralyzed from a tumor on her spinal column. In spite of everything we did on an emergency basis, she did not and will not recover from her paralysis. I made it clear to her that there was no other reasonable treatment for her progressive cancer. Later, after all of this tragic news had had time to sink in, I walked into her room and asked her how she was doing. "I'll be fine," she said. When I had finished talking with her and began to leave, she said, "It'll be all right, Dr. Weir. God is good."

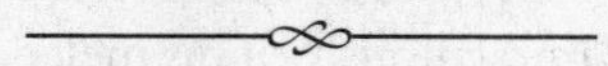

These proclamations by two women in the midst of suffering are lights that cannot be overcome by the dark cries of those who from a distance would say, "A good and powerful God would never let her suffer." These women in their suffering were satisfied with God. They each found their way to the presence of God, and somehow the questions were no longer relevant. Knowing God brought the realization that God can be trusted. Knowing God, they accepted their inability to understand his way while at the same time they accepted his love and power. Isaiah told the exiled people in Babylon, "'For my thoughts are not your thoughts, neither are your ways my ways,' declares the Lord. 'As the heavens are higher than the earth, so are my ways higher than your ways and my thoughts than your thoughts'" (Isa. 55:8–9).

The answer to the question "Why?" comes in knowing God.

The answer to the question "Why?" comes in knowing God. When I am with him, I realize who he is; I know that his purpose is greater, more important, and better for me than a release from my suffering. I know that being with him in suffering is better than being without him in comfort. In spite of our suffering, even if that suffering leads to death, we can say with David, "Let him do to me whatever seems good to him" (2 Sam. 15:26). And even if there is no deliverance, we can say with Jesus, "Father, into your hands I commit my spirit" (Luke 23:46).

GOD IS FAITHFUL

Whatever the answers to our questions, if we want peace within our illness, we must rest upon the faithfulness of God. It was true in the Bible. It is true in our lives.

David was delivered from his son Absalom. God was faithful.

Daniel was thrown into the lions' den. The next morning the king pulled him out. Not a lion's tooth had touched him. God was faithful.

William was cured miraculously of his melanoma. God was faithful.

God is faithful even if we are not healed. Ralph and Linda Bethea were missionaries in Kenya. One night they were driving from Mombassa to Nairobi. An injured man lay in the road; or so they thought. Ralph stopped the car to help, and a group of bandits crawled over the rocks and attacked. Linda got out of the car and was struck across the head. Ralph drove the bandits off, then Linda died in his arms. Was God faithful?

Stephen served poor widows and preached the Word of God. The crowd took him to the edge of the city and stoned him until he died. Was God faithful?

Ellen McCall spent her life for the Lord and died of cancer. Was God faithful?

Each of these succumbed to their tragedies, but *each claimed God was faithful*. Who am I to say they were mistaken?

You and I will someday die as well. Is God faithful?

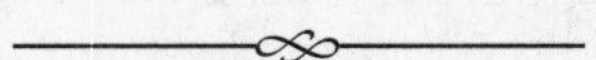

God is faithful. Some of us suffer now; some of us suffer later; all of us suffer someday. Deliverance from one time of suffering is not a test of God's faithfulness, because God's purpose is to deliver us from all suffering. The working out of that purpose is far beyond our ability to understand. But we can know him. And when we know him—the one who lived and died and rose again and prepares a place for us to live with him forever, the one who sees, who loves, and who has the power of the resurrection—we can crawl into his arms, take the question "Why?" and lay it aside until the day when we sit and chat with him in eternity.

NINE

Choose to Keep Praying

The way we seek God's presence most directly is through prayer. That's certainly been true in my own life. I was very young the first time I experienced God's answer to prayer. I don't remember it; I only remember being told about it. I have mentioned this story before, but let me tell you the details. I was less than one year old when my parents realized I was different. I did not eat well, and my motor skills did not develop as they had in my older sister by the same age. My father is a doctor, so he had the inside track to excellent care. Appropriate studies were performed, and my brain was found to be degenerating, leaving my skull full of fluid.

Doctors initiated aggressive measures to reverse the process with shunts, but these were not effective. My parents were told to place me in an institution and expect me to spend my life as a vegetable. They had little hope, but they had a lot of love for me and decided to care for me themselves.

My Aunt Eunice was not scientific enough to accept the neurosurgeon's pronouncement. She carried me to her church, where I was anointed with oil. Christians of faith prayed for my healing. The disease resolved, and my brain has been functioning fairly well ever since.

Though I cannot remember the event, I am confident that God used the prayers and faith of those members of that small church as a channel for his power to heal me. Many times since, I have recorded incidents in which God issued his power through human prayer to provide healing, relief, or guidance to accomplish impossible desires. When such happens, most people of faith say, "God answers prayer."

I have had many other experiences in my life when that which I desired and prayed for earnestly did not occur. All of us face tragedies in our future. All of us will die someday, even as someone is praying earnestly for us to live. Our experience thus seems to say, "God answers prayers but not always."

In his book *Of Human Bondage,* Somerset Maugham describes a young man with a great desire. Philip Carey was a boy with a club foot. He hated it. All the kids at school made fun of him. One day he read the words of Jesus, "If you have faith, and doubt not . . . you shall say to the mountain, 'Be thou removed, and be thou cast in the sea; it shall be done.'" A few nights later, Philip prayed with all his heart that his foot would be healed. He went to sleep dreaming of running and playing with the other boys. When he awakened in the morning, he was excited and grateful that he had been healed; but when he reached to touch his foot, he found it unchanged. He asked his minister uncle what it meant if you prayed in faith for something to happen and it didn't come to pass. His uncle told him that meant he had not enough faith. So he gave God twenty more days, revving up his faith the entire time. Still the foot remained crippled. "I suppose no one ever has faith enough," Philip said. I don't believe he ever prayed again.[1]

In earlier chapters we have already suggested that God is capable of providing for us that which we desire (see Eph. 3:20). We have already stated that God loves us as his own children when we approach him in prayer (see Matt. 7:7–11). What then can we do with prayers that seem to go unanswered? Are there reasons that sometimes our great desires carried to God and placed in his hands are denied?

Of course, there are many reasons we might not see God move in the way we ask. Some of these reasons are in God's hands and must be left there. But others are in our hands, and we should consider whether a change in our lives might allow us to better see God's power. Let me mention some areas in which you might choose to change in a way that could transform your prayers into avenues for God's power.

BROKEN RELATIONSHIPS

Often I have seen patients struggle to find God but fail because of a relationship that has been tormenting their life and needs to be mended.

> And when you stand praying, if you hold anything against anyone, forgive him, so that your Father in heaven may forgive you your sins.
>
> —MARK 11:25

> Therefore, if you are offering your gift at the altar and there remember that your brother has something against you, leave your gift there in front of the altar. First go and be reconciled to your brother; then come and offer your gift.
>
> —MATTHEW 5:23–24

I remember a woman with breast cancer that had spread to her spine. This patient had been consistently noncompliant in her care, suspicious, and angry. One day I saw her sitting in our chemotherapy room talking to my nurse, Robbie, and crying. Later I asked Robbie why she was crying. "She has a sister who she has not spoken to for five years, and she thinks she may never see her again. I told her to call her today and change it now." The patient did contact her sister, and for the last year of her life there was a peace about her living and a change in her relationship with us that I would never have thought possible.

God says, "When you come to me with a request or in worship, if you hold anything against your brother or he against you, set it straight first; then I will work with you." Ask yourself: Is there a relationship I can correct before I go to God? Is there someone who has wronged me whom I need to forgive? Is there someone I have wronged with whom I have to work to make it right? God says, "I will not deal with you in a vacuum. I will relate to you dependent to some degree on how you relate to other people."

We've got to heal broken relationships on earth if we wish to see fully his power from heaven. The truth is, one of the greatest manifestations of his power and one of the greatest answers to unspoken prayer in your life would be to heal the broken relationship between you and someone you love. Your feet, your hands, your lips, and his power can do it.

DISOBEDIENCE

We know that sometimes there is sin in our lives that stands as a barrier to our communication with the Father.

> Your iniquities have separated you from your God; your sins have hidden his face from you, so that he will not hear.
>
> —ISAIAH 59:2

> [We] receive from him anything we ask, because we obey his commands and do what pleases him.
>
> —1 JOHN 3:22

When a prayer seems unanswered, it's time to ask if there is a sin I need to clear from my life. Is there a command from God that I am not obeying? I have told of my wife Becky's sickness with her second pregnancy. When we thought she might die, we planned to abort the child as a last-chance effort to save Becky's life. We continued to pray for deliverance from God even as we pursued the possibility of abortion. It was only when we refused the abortion *regardless of Becky's health* that God answered our prayer and healed her sickness. Disobedience and sin can plug the pipeline of God's power. We certainly should look at our lives as we beg for deliverance and clear the sin before we can expect an answer.

Mike did. He was a patient of mine with brain cancer. Mike told me that the first thing he did when he found out he was seriously ill was to look for sin in his life that might interfere with God's will in the midst of his illness. He discovered that he was neglecting his family by working too hard. He corrected that sin and then felt confident he could communicate with the Father. God clearly spoke to Mike and did an amazing work in bringing him through that illness. If we can confess our sin, change our behavior, and let the blood of Christ cleanse us, some of us might be healed from the sickness that accompanies us through life. And even if we are not healed, with the sin out of our lives, we at least can walk through life hand-in-hand with the God who knows the way to eternity.

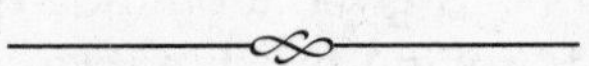

We must be careful, however, with this understanding of our need for forgiveness. We must not take the leap from sin as an obstruction to prayer all the way to sin as the cause of our suffering. My experience as an oncologist for many people of faith is that rarely have I found sin to be the major problem that prevents God from healing through prayer. Most people are not sick as a direct result of their personal sin and are not healed simply because they pray. We need to be careful that we don't blame our individual sickness on our individual sin and our lack of healing on our individual disobedience. We all have sinned, but there is a cross in the heart of God that seeks to save, not to punish. Too many people feel that God is punishing them with their illness. I believe this is rarely the case. As we seek forgiveness for the sin in our lives, we need to remember that our God is a God of love and mercy, a God who does not wish his children to suffer and die.

Most people are not sick as a result of their sin and are not healed simply because they pray.

DISTANCE FROM THE FATHER

Although sin in our lives will at times inhibit God's power, sometimes we make the mistake of believing that the answer to our prayers is solely dependent on the score we achieve, adding up our obedience and subtracting our sin. God has always made it clear that the most important aspect of our lives is not our score but our relationship with him.

> You may ask me for anything in my name, and I will do it.
>
> —JOHN 14:14

> If you remain in me and my words remain in you, ask whatever you wish, and it will be given you.
>
> —JOHN 15:7

Let me tell you a story: Evelyn sat on the front porch, angry at life for the loneliness it had brought her, but relaxed in the gentle breeze and pastoral scene before her. All she had left was her farm, with its rolling pastures and horses that would take off and run with the wind whenever they pleased. She was not old, but she was beaten down by a life that had taken her husband in death when she was young and then drove her son away to work in the city when he was less than twenty. It had been forty years since he left, and never a word after "Good-bye, Mom." She once had friends, but she had driven them all away except Nate Cawthorne, a crusty old widower who refused to give up on her. Don't reckon he had any thoughts of elderly romance, but he kept being a friend when she needed a friend, even when she had tried her best to turn him away. Every Saturday he would come and sit on her porch and look out over the pastures with her. He'd sit there without a word for thirty minutes, just looking off like she did, then finally break the silence with something he noticed in a particular horse's stride or new shade of color in an autumn tree. They would gradually build up a conversation, and somehow he would figure out something she needed each visit, such that the next week she'd see him fixing a fence or patching the roof without her ever asking or expecting.

Now he was gone too—buried two years—the only friend she had known in a lonely world. She had sort of expected it, since life was like that anyway. The good thing was that she had lost everyone that mattered now, and she could live in peace without human intrusions.

She saw the man coming over the rise in the distance. He was walking slowly with a slight limp. He looked fairly young as he approached, maybe thirty or forty, and seemed he'd had a hard life by the weathered skin and wasted temples. He reminded her of someone, but whom she did not know. He didn't speak until he had stopped in the dirt at the edge of the porch, then took off his hat and sort of stuttered, "I sure am hungry, ma'am, and would work for food today if you like," he said.

The anger welled up inside of her. Here she was all alone, caring for herself, and here comes a bum off the road wanting a handout. Just another insult from life.

"I don't know who sent you up here looking for a handout, but you've come to the wrong place. Get on down the road and take your begging to people that care," she said, leaning forward in her rocker with granite in her face.

He lowered his head, replaced his hat, and turned to go, but he stopped and turned back and spoke again with his eyes down, "They've already turned me away. I've got nowhere else to go. I just got out of the state prison and came home hoping to get started again, but no one wants me around. My dad mentioned you a few times in his letters; said your heart was bigger than most folks' even though you buried it pretty deep. I came to you last, cause I never asked for help from a woman before. He said I could count on you. I know it's my fault I've got no place to go, and I ain't worth much, but a man tries to keep living even when he don't deserve to."

She leaned back in her chair and looked out over her pastures. Something had spooked the horse, and he was galloping over the second rise; or maybe he'd just wanted to feel the wind in his face.

"I don't know your father, nor nobody's father," she said, still looking off. "He wrote you about some other lady. I got no need for you, and I don't want you here. I'm sorry you've got your troubles, but they are nothing to me. Get off my land and leave me alone."

She didn't see the anger rise in his face or see him reach into his pocket. But she looked again because of the ice in his voice and saw the gun in his hand.

"I didn't plan to do this, lady, but I'm hungry and I've got to eat," he said, "so get up out of that chair and get me some food!"

She felt a brief twinge of fear, but it passed quickly. She sighed and leaned back in her chair. "Go ahead and shoot," she said. "Life's not worth much anyway."

His face turned beet red as he threw the gun against the wall of the house beside her. The noise made her jump a bit. He turned away again and began to limp down the gravel drive. As he did, she noticed his left hand. She had not seen it earlier, but the ring finger was shorter than the rest. She had known a hand like that before.

"Who's your father?" she demanded.

"His name was Nate Cawthorne," he replied. "He's been dead awhile, before I came out of jail."

"He was a good man," she said. "I reckon I do have some work around here for you. That fence hasn't been mended since he died. I got a spare room you can stay in for a few days. Dinner will be ready at six o'clock. Tools are in the shed."

Young Nate Cawthorne brushed the dusty tears from his eyes with a ragged sleeve as he limped to the shed to start his work.

God doesn't answer our prayers because we are good enough. He doesn't answer our prayers because we've followed the rules. And he doesn't reject our prayers because we've broken the rules. We can't force God to do what we want by showing him our actions or our faith or his promises. He doesn't answer our prayers because of who we are. He answers our prayers because he loves us, because of whom we know and whose we are. God answers our prayers because of our relationship with him, and those of us who are Christians believe that that relationship comes through Jesus Christ.

The one to whom you pray will become more important to you than the prayers.

How close are you to the Son of God? Is the presence of the Christ real in your life? As you look ahead toward your suffering and face great needs and great desires, you need to spend time with him through whom your prayers can be answered. You will discover that the one to whom you pray becomes more important to you than the prayers themselves.

Wrong Motives

Sometimes God does not move in the direction we want him to move because our motives are self-centered rather than God-centered.

"You want something but don't get it. You kill and covet, but you cannot have what you want. You quarrel and you fight. You do not have, because you do not ask God. When you ask, you do not receive, because you ask with wrong motives, that you may spend what you get on your pleasures" (James 4:2–3).

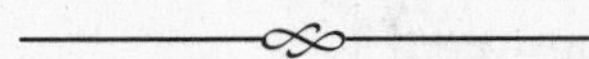

As a father, I love my three children, and it is wonderful to see the happiness on their faces when I give them something they really want. I probably get more joy from that than they do. But I can't stand it and even get angry at times when we walk into a store for a baseball and Bowen demands a new glove, a new bat, roller blades, a .22 rifle, and a six-inch hunting knife. We went to the store because we needed the ball, but Bowen gets angry and pouts and ruins the fun we were going to have because he does not get all the things he wants. The point of the trip to the store was to obtain something we needed to allow us to have a great day together. The other stuff he wanted was surplus, a distraction.

What stuff do we ask God for? Perhaps some of the things we desire most are really surplus and distractions. God, as a loving Father, hears and wants to please us. But what he wants most is to give us what is necessary to have a great day with him and a great life forever with him. He wants the same for those we love as well. As you look at the difficulties in your future, what do you need in order to strengthen your relationship with God, to strengthen your relationship with those you love, and to strengthen God's relationship with those you love? Pray for those things, and expect an answer. Don't be surprised if the answer to those prayers relieves your pain and loneliness more than any drug a doctor can prescribe.

Misunderstood Answers

Sometimes we don't recognize God's answer when we see it because we expect something different. The apostle Paul said of his suffering, "Three times I pleaded with the Lord to take it away from me. But he said to me, 'My grace is sufficient for you, for my power is made perfect in weakness'" (2 Cor. 12:8–9).

A few years ago Garth Brooks came out with a song entitled "Unanswered Prayers." In it he describes his high school sweetheart and related how he had prayed to God that their love would last forever. The love didn't last, and some years later he was attending a high school reunion with the wife he truly loved. Here comes his high school sweetheart. He looks at her and then looks at his wife and thanks God that his high school prayer was not answered.[2]

In his book *The Meaning of Prayer,* Harry Emerson Fosdick says that we sometimes miss God's answer to prayer because "if God granted the form of our petition, he would deny the substance of our desire."[3] Paul's greatest desire was to draw close to Christ and to bring all men unto him. God refused Paul's petition to relieve his suffering and, in doing so, manifested his power in Paul's weakness, thus granting Paul's greatest desire.

St. Augustine, in his *Confessions,* relates the torment his mother went through before he accepted the lordship of Christ. Augustine decided to leave his home and mother for Italy to broaden his horizons. His mother was frantic over the thought of his absence from her influence. She was certain that her libertine son would never find Christ in the libertine environment of Italy. She prayed all night at a seaside chapel on the evening before his departure, asking God to keep him home, but Augustine sailed on. It was in Italy that Augustine came to accept Christ as Savior. In a later prayer, Augustine relates his understanding of the event: "Thou in the depth of Thy counsels, hearing the main point of her desire, regardest not what she asked, that Thou mightest make me what she ever desired."[4]

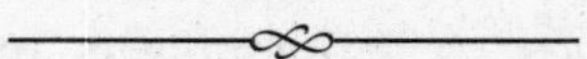

As you look into your future toward real difficulties, there will come to you many needs and desires not only for yourself but also for those who will be affected by what you are going through. Timing is urgent to you. You may know exactly what needs to be done to make it all work out. You throw your requests to God, but his answer doesn't come within your timetable, or the answer seems to be "no," or he doesn't even seem to hear you. You must understand that God's ways are not your ways; they are better for you and those you love than your ways. You need to accept that sometimes what seems to be a denial is in fact a "Yes, I'll take care of that, but it's better to do it in a different way. Trust me. I love you."

LACK OF TRUST

We may not see God act because we do not trust him to do so.

> Therefore I tell you, whatever you ask for in prayer, believe that you have received it, and it will be yours.
>
> —MARK 11:24

One of my nurses loves azaleas, but she never has grown them. We were talking on rounds the other day about the unusual weather in Memphis, which is extraordinary in its fickleness, particularly during winter. We may experience an ice storm one week in February, then the next week sunny skies in the mid-seventies, then ice again. It makes an interesting winter, but it confuses the plants. Often the flowers, particularly azaleas, will be fooled into budding, only to be wiped out by a hard freeze, leaving few flowers for the spring. This particular nurse refuses to plant azaleas because she fears they will die or fail to bloom in the spring. Consequently, she never enjoys beautiful blossoms except at a distance in other people's yards. She never has azalea blossoms because she doesn't trust them to grow safely.

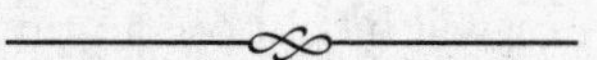

We will rarely see God answer prayer if we don't trust him to answer our prayers. Not only must we believe in our minds that God will answer, but we must work out that expectancy in our lives. We have to plant the azaleas. For some reason, God has developed a pipeline for his power with a valve at our end that must be opened. Faith is the knob that opens the pipeline of God's power. Have you turned the knob in your life? Do you trust that God can do all things in your situation? If not, you may be blocking the flow of his power to act in your life in ways you can't even imagine.

We must be careful. Some people believe more in faith than they do in God. The valve on our end is only a valve. It is God who sends the power where he wills in his love and wisdom. Just because we open the valve with our faith does not mean that we will witness his power accomplish what we wish. However, we will rarely witness his power if we do not trust him to act in our lives.

OUTSIDE OF GOD'S WILL

We also need to accept the truth that many times God does not move the way we ask him because some things are simply not God's will.

> This is the confidence we have in approaching God:
> that if we ask anything *according to his will,* he hears us.
>
> —1 JOHN 5:14 (ITALICS MINE)

An earnest prayer for something we feel is worthy and important might not be answered because it is outside of God's purpose. Each of us will come to times in our lives when our desire does not agree with his plan. When this happens, we must realize that God's action in our lives does not begin with his plan. God's action in our lives always begins with his love: "God is love" (1 John 4:8). God's action originates in love, then passes through omniscience. God told the exiled children of Israel, "As the heavens are higher than the earth, so are my ways higher than your ways and my thoughts higher than your thoughts" (Isa. 55:9). God's plan flows from his love for us and is formulated within his understanding of us. He chooses not to do anything that contradicts his love for mankind, nor will he choose an unwise course. In his love and wisdom, we see him work in our lives and sometimes, to our disappointment, that work is not what we desire.

My son, Bowen, is at the age when he is not yet inhibited in asking for what he wants. Today there were a number of requests: he asked for a jet ski, a horse, and a Hummer—all of which he felt he truly needed. When I said "no" to each, he became somber and withdrew from me for a while. Later he came back and snuggled up in my arms as Becky drove me to the airport. He was unhappy with me for not accommodating his desires, but he eventually surrendered to his trust of me based on our years together and his desire to be with the father he loves.

When the doctor hands you bad news, you may beg God to somehow help you avoid the harsh reality. If it seems your request is being denied, do not play the part of the child who never returns to the Father's arms because of your disappointment. Eventually come to accept that God has a plan for your life, and for mankind, that is wiser and more loving than your own. Eventually realize that you can trust your life and the lives of those you love to his plan. Eventually push aside your resentment and crawl back into the arms of the one you love, the one who died for you, and the only one who can carry you into eternity.

TEN

Choose Real Value

In the beautiful lyrics to his song "Vincent," Don McLean describes the life, work, and death of Vincent Van Gogh, depicting Van Gogh's despair over the world's indifference to his art.[1] During Van Gogh's lifetime, the public held little regard for his paintings, but now their value is extraordinary, selling regularly for more than a million dollars. One day, feeling desperate over his lack of self-worth, Van Gogh shot himself in the chest and died in his brother's arms. Neither he nor the world at that time understood the value of his existence.

How do you decide what is of value in your own life? Do you live your life focused on the right things? If you are now looking toward a difficult future, it is critical that you decide what you should hold on to while you live out the rest of your life.

In Luke 12:16–21, Jesus tells us a story about values. If he told it today, it might go something like this:

> Ten more minutes and it will be five o'clock. Ten more minutes and I will have made it! That has to be the reason for this meeting. I'm the only one capable of the position, and he asked me to meet with him at

five, and he smiled when he said it. I've finally made it! With the job come stock options, and with the stock options I retire at fifty.

Finally I'll be able to spend the time with Britt Jr. that I've been wanting to spend. His senior year in high school, and I'll finally get to his ball games. Oh, I wish I had had some time with Rachel when she was home. Poor thing, will she ever be happy? I'll start exercising now so I can enjoy the travel (and look good in Acapulco).

Janice needs to work out too if I'm going to walk those beaches with her. She's got a belly just like her mother did. What if she stays fat? I need to get her looking good again. I've been noticing too many other women lately; I've got to stop that. But, man, Sandra looks good. She smells like heaven, and she looks at me with those eyes that say, "We're more than just coworkers, and you know it." When she touches me, I feel like a college junior again at homecoming in the football stands, keeping warm and thinking of later. What am I going to do about her? If I get any closer, I won't be able to stop, and I don't want to stop. I'll work it out.

Whatever happens, I'd never leave Janice while Britt Jr. is still at home. Man, I wish I could make his game tonight, but after this meeting I need to come back to the office and prove I'm as good as the boss thinks I am. Janice will go to Britt Jr.'s game. She always does. Maybe we can get away this weekend to our cabin at the lake and make up for lost time. Dang, I've got to meet with my investment broker on Saturday. If I can just get a bonus, that will put me over $1,000,000 in my portfolio. Then, with the stock options!

"Hello, Britt Warner here, what can I do for you? . . . What do you mean, Doc? You said I was in top shape when I left your office. . . . What's wrong with my blood? Tell me now, Doc; I've got a big meeting in five minutes that will guarantee me everything. I can't

> wait to discuss it tomorrow! . . . Leukemia? What does that mean? How long will I be off work? . . . You can't do this to me!"

Jesus finished his story two thousand years ago with the statement, "You fool! This very night your life will be demanded from you. Then who will get what you have prepared for yourself?" (Luke 12:20).

One could say that leukemia is a rare disorder and that we should not base decisions in our lives on unlikely tragedies. I've treated more than a hundred patients with leukemia who felt this way until their leukemia was discovered. Then there is breast cancer, a heart attack, stroke, corporate restructuring, and divorce. As the list grows, an unlikely tragedy in life becomes a common interruption in plans that each of us must face someday. The point of the story is not that we should live our lives expecting tragedy. The point is to examine our value system and weigh it against the realities of life.

Our value system is naturally linked to our concept of time on earth and an expectancy of a life of seventy-some years. If this is the way we view our life on earth, with nothing more after death, we very rationally place the greatest value in our lives on those things that bring us pleasure during our lifetime. Unfortunately, this leads to two tragic consequences:

1. When we are faced with the end of our life on earth, all that we have gathered and valued can help us only as memories, and even those memories are gone when death closes our eyes.
2. Our hearts are tied to that which we value. When we see death approaching or if the doctor's bad news changes our lives in drastic ways, we face the tearing away of all that we value, and with that comes despair.

Jesus understood this when he said, "Do not store up for yourselves treasures on earth, where moth and rust destroy, and where thieves break in and steal. But store up for yourselves treasures in heaven, where moth and rust do not destroy, and where thieves do not break in and steal. *For where your treasure is, there your heart will be also*" (Matt. 6:19–20, italics mine).

When the doctor gives you bad news, it is the tearing away of the things of the heart that brings the despair. Catherine can never do gymnastics again after breaking her back. A wonderful symphony violinist I know can no longer read music after lung surgery led to a stroke. Is it possible to develop a value system in which our hearts are not dependent on things that vanish when an illness steals from us that which we most cherish?

We were placed on this earth with the privilege and responsibility to choose what we value. Some people choose to value Van Gogh's paintings. Some choose to value money. Others choose to value physical affection. In a popular movie, one man who valued physical affection offered another man, who valued money, $1 million to borrow his beautiful wife for one night. I missed the movie and don't know how it ended. But how it ended isn't important. What is important is to understand Jesus' message: that this is a life where neither money nor physical attraction lasts forever.

A recent article in our local newspaper told the story of a British factory worker named Ernie who won a lottery prize worth $18.6 million. Ernie died after a twenty-month binge on cigarettes, alcohol, and take-out food. He ignored all advice to quit drinking and smoking and died in his luxury bungalow at 310 pounds. A family friend said, "Poor old Ernie is proof you can't take it with you."

We often realize the truth of that statement only when we face death. It is then that we can grasp the understanding of life about which Omar Khayyam wrote:

> The Worldly Hope men set their hearts upon
> Turns ashes—or it prospers; and anon,
> Like snow upon the Desert's dusty face,
> Lighting a little hour or two—is gone.[2]

We can face life with the understanding and despair of Omar Khayyam. Or we can ignore the truth that earthly treasures are temporary. Or we can learn to value treasure that outlasts the grave and maintains its value in the face of serious health changes.

Murray Alexander is a wealthy retired farmer from the delta of Mississippi, a region of flat, rich soil carried there over the centuries by the Mississippi River. He came to me two years ago with an impossible situation. Six months prior to our meeting, he had had a kidney removed for cancer. Now he had two spots that looked like cancer in his liver. We took biopsies of them and confirmed the suspicion. We used our best science and prayers and put him through a terrible course of therapy with a drug called Interleukin 2, resulting in fevers, swelling, rashes, severe weakness, and weight loss. The lesions on the liver remained stable. There was no evidence of other cancer, so he was taken to surgery. All cancerous tissue at the time of surgery was found to be destroyed.

Suffering and the threat of death with God beside you are more valuable than a comfortable life without him.

It has been over a year now since the last surgery, and Mr. Alexander is just now recovering all of his strength. There is still no evidence of cancer. He related to me in a recent office visit, "When I learned about the cancer in my liver, a verse came into my mind, 'My peace I leave with you.' I never prayed for healing, because I didn't know if it was his best will. But God's peace has never left me. And if I could trade the last two years of suffering for two years of health, I would never do it." This was not the voice of a fanatic or a confused, sick man. Mr. Alexander had discovered a great mystery: real suffering and the threat of death with God beside you are more valuable than a comfortable life without him.

What do you look for when you walk through your world? Do you strain your neck seeking pleasures that will satisfy your personal desires? Or do you notice a mighty and loving Father gathering a broken world into his arms? Do you have a vision for the eternal when you walk through this world?

When we see only the material and concrete things of this world, we are motivated to acquire what we see. We move through life seeking what we think will make us happy but find great gaps in our satisfaction between our successes. And then we die.

In John 6:27 Jesus noted the problem of fulfilling satisfaction with the pleasures of this world: it all spoils. Either the things we acquire will spoil through rust, age, and decay, or our desire for them will spoil. Everything in this world that we acquire to satisfy our personal senses will eventually diminish in appeal, and we will be driven to seek something new, something fresh and unspoiled. Then, in facing death, anything in this world that still satisfies us is torn from our grasp.

Jesus did not warn us of this to depress us. He wants us to face the truth because there is something better. He tells us there is something more satisfying now, something that will not diminish in its appeal, something eternal, something that will last forever, something that he will give you.

Jesus says, "Choose God instead of earthly treasures. He will not disappoint you now, and he will not disappoint you at death."

How well have you chosen your treasures?

Jesus once stood on a hillside in Galilee and explained to his disciples how radically different our lives would be if we chose God as our treasure. In words we now know as the Beatitudes, he began by saying, "Blessed are the poor in spirit, for theirs is the kingdom of heaven" (Matt. 5:3). William Barclay, in his commentary, restates this Beatitude, "Blessed is the man who has realized his own utter helplessness, and who has put his whole trust in God."[3]

Facing serious illness or death is a very effective means of shaking our confidence, making us "poor in spirit." Not many of us can face death and say, "I've got it figured out, and I can handle it." I did know a patient who repaired Porsches, spoke five languages, took echinacea, and refused to accept God. God never made much sense to him. He is one of the very few people I've met who maintained his confidence in his own ability to fix things right up to his death. You may be the same. But most of us do not go so confidently into the night of serious illness or death. Most of us cry out, "I am not able to face this on my own! God, help me!" When we are thus "poor in spirit," we finally seek God, and in seeking him, we find him, and the kingdom of heaven can be ours.

The Beatitudes continue, "Blessed are those who mourn, for they will be comforted" (Matt. 5:4). Most of us can remember being brokenhearted as a child over the loss of something dear to us. (For my son at age ten, it was a motorized truck that was run over by an aggressive teenager in a white van.) Afterward we remember crawling into our mother's or father's lap and feeling the comfort of their arms. When we look back on the event, the comfort of those arms fills our heart with a joy that overwhelms the painful memory of the loss. The pain of the loss was nothing compared to the comfort of our mother's or father's arms. Do you want to feel the arms of God? If in your tears you follow him, he promises that you will be comforted.

Jesus continued, "Blessed are the meek, for they will inherit the earth" (Matt. 5:5). Meek is not weak. The meek are those who renounce their own personal rights for the sake of others and for God. Jesus had rights that came with being God. He gave them up when he walked the earth and died on a cross. We all feel that we have personal rights as well: the right to family, to health, to control of our own affairs, to watch our children grow, to a good life if we work hard. The doctor's bad news ignores our personal rights, takes them away, and pays for them with nothingness. Jesus says, "Don't wait until some tragic health problem steals from you what you think you deserve. Give up your personal rights now in pursuit of me, and instead of nothingness, you will inherit the earth."

There is great comfort in the Beatitudes for those who trust in God. When we face illness and death, we can look to what Jesus promised as he sat on that mountainside teaching the crowd that day so long ago. When we mourn, we will be comforted. He promised. He keeps his promises.

> You have filled my heart with greater joy
> than when their grain and new wine abound.
> I will lie down and sleep in peace,
> for you alone, O Lord,
> make me dwell in safety.
>
> —PSALM 4:7–8

As you face the doctor's bad news, you can choose how you view the world. Will you choose to view time as eternal? Will you choose to view life as spiritual as well as physical? Will you choose to see God as good? Will you choose to value your relationship with him more than the things of the world? Even if your body and dreams are broken, it is possible to find greater value in your life ahead than you have known in the years of health gone by.

ELEVEN

Choose to Pursue Joy

Rebecca has lung cancer with little time to live. The other day I asked her, "Can you tell me something good that has happened to you since I saw you last?" She answered, "Oh, lots of good things have happened. My children were home this weekend, and we were able to get a number of things discussed that we needed to because of my illness, like who should get what when I am gone. My kids were kind of fun about it. There was some stuff I like a lot that none of them want. We were trying to divide it up. I said, 'Please, somebody take this,' and they would say to each other, 'Why don't you take that.'"

She told me how her grandchildren came over. One of them had a friend who asked Rebecca what had happened to her hair. She told the youngster, "Well, I was sick and the doctor gave me some medicines that made me better but made by hair go away." The little boy then asked, "Where did your hair go?" She told him that she had saved the hair she had lost. He then said, "Well, get some water, put it on the hair, then pat it on your head, and it will stay." Rebecca laughed at the child's common sense, and her day was better.

Rebecca walked into my room that day with end-stage cancer but left with joy and the feeling that life is worth living. What brings joy to people's lives when these lives are filled with fear and pain? I have learned that joy will not always put an arm around our shoulders, but there are steps we can take to bring it back, and when we are broken, it is often the return of joy that makes life worth living again.

Seek the Joyful Event

Robert was old and wasted from two cancers when I sat with him, but he was looking forward to the Fourth of July celebration. No longer was he the cook, but there would be ribs, pork shoulders, and sausage on the grill, and he could watch, talk with, and listen to all of his relatives. He could smile in spite of his cancers because the joy of the event was ahead. Death was somewhere further down the road.

> *List things you've always wanted to do, then walk through the rest of life checking them off as you do them.*

Many of us tend to withdraw and lick our wounds when we know death is in our visible future or when sickness keeps us from pleasures we knew before. We cannot imagine joy again in our lives. It doesn't have to be that way. You may not be able to force yourself to feel happy again, but you can force yourselves to plan events that will drag joy back into your life. Rather than curling up in a corner until the rest of life passes, sit at a desk and list the things you've always wanted to do, then walk through the rest of life checking off the possibilities as you do them.

Spend Time with Those You Love

A young woman in our community had suffered for many years with a blood disorder. The disorder was changing rapidly into an uncontrollable process. She was ill but very much wished to travel on a vacation with her husband and eight-year-old child. She seemed healthy enough to handle the trip, so they left for Hawaii. She and her husband knew this might be their last vacation together. They had a great time during the first week of their vacation, but then she developed lung and heart problems. She died in Hawaii. Although she is gone, and her parting is tragic for all of us, she lived her last days filled with joy and shared them with those she loved.

Rather than running from people when illness overtakes you, you need to seek them—selectively. There may not be enough time left for shallow relationships. Choose the people you really wish to be with. Devote your time to sharing life with each of them. Joy will come as you sit beside the ones you love.

Borrow the Joy of Those You Love

If you can't find joy in your own situation, borrow joy from those you love. How about watching your grandson score the winning soccer goal and letting the smile on his face shape your own? How about attending your brother's birthday celebration and focusing on the joy you wish for him? His joy will become your own. You might even *cause* joyful things to happen to those you love, then let that joy fill your days. A patient of mine with breast cancer planned a cruise for her grown daughters and their husbands. She traveled with them, in spite of her discomfort, and not only enjoyed their company but was blessed by the joy the cruise brought into their lives. Even in her suffering she could bring joy to others and then participate in that joy.

Draw Close to Your Greatest Friend—God

The only friend who will hold your hand all the way through the tough things of life and then through the gates of death is God. Murray Alexander, whom I quoted earlier, understood. "I did not pray that God would heal me, because I did not know if that was his will. I prayed instead that he would be with me, and he has never left me." Jesus said as he approached his own death, "I am the vine; you are the branches.... As the Father has loved me, so have I loved you. Now remain in my love.... I have told you this so that my joy may be in you and that your joy may be complete" (John 15:5–11).

While in prison near the end of his life, Paul wrote to the church at Philippi, "Rejoice in the Lord always. I will say it again: Rejoice! Let your gentleness be evident to all. The Lord is near. Do not be anxious about anything, but in everything, by prayer and petition, with thanksgiving, present your requests to God. And the peace of God, which transcends all understanding, will guard your hearts and your minds in Christ Jesus" (Phil. 4:4–7). Paul, facing his own death, says we can be full of joy, not because of the suffering, but because God is near and his very presence will bring joy into our lives.

Seek him as you face your suffering. Dedicate time to pray, time to read his Word, time to sit, and time to listen for his voice. The joy you feel as you face your difficulties will become greater the closer you are to the one who rules eternity.

Find Hope

Hope is looking forward toward something or someone who will bring us joy. Hope lets us borrow joy from the future to use now. Hope might be found in the planned events or planned encounters that we have already mentioned, but hope can also be found in events beyond the grave. Matthew is a seventy-two-year-old patient of mine with colon cancer that has spread to the liver. He recently failed all standard therapy for his condition and chose to live out his life without experimental therapy. With a calm smile he said to me, "I am not worried about death. I know death is a doorway to heaven. I've got my mother, father, and four brothers there waiting to greet me." His hope in that reunion beyond the grave is bringing joy to him as he walks toward the grave. Paul wrote of this reunion in his letter to the Thessalonian church: "For the Lord himself will come down from heaven, with a loud command, with the voice of the archangel and with the trumpet call of God, and the dead in Christ will rise first. After that, we who are still alive and are left will be caught up together with them in the clouds to meet the Lord in the air. And so we will be with the Lord forever" (1 Thess. 4:16–17).

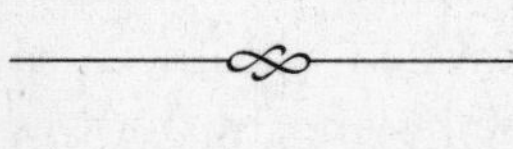

The joy you feel as you face your difficulties will become greater the closer you are to the one who rules eternity.

Life is tough to live without joy, and health tragedies drain that joy from our lives and make us die inside long before we cease to breathe. But this need not happen. In the face of suffering, you can actively pursue joy. You can plan events and encounters now that will fill your life with joy. You can borrow the joy of others if you are willing to focus on their happiness rather than your own grief. You can act to increase their happiness, and this will increase your joy. You can hope, not as a wishful thought but as a firm expectation, for wonderful people and events ahead, not only in this world but at the feet of our Father in eternity.

Look for the Good

Pollyanna got a bad rap. She's the girl who looked for the silver lining in every cloud, even to the point of finding something good in breaking her back. Her name has actually developed into an accusation describing a person who is sickeningly cheerful about their own or someone else's misery. But Pollyanna was right. There is some good within everything that happens, no matter how severe the event, including death and serious illness. How we tolerate a difficult situation in part depends on whether we discover the good within it.

How we tolerate difficulty depends in part on whether we discover the good within it.

The other day at a family lunch, Aunt Letta Ree told a story about her young granddaughter, Alex. Letta Ree was attempting to plant a seed of etiquette within the youngster, so she planned a tea party in which Alex would invite her friends, dress up, and serve the refreshments. Alex was excited about the idea and did a beautiful job with all of it, following her grandmother's instructions precisely. After serving the tea, little Alex sat down and led the conversation, telling the following story:

"Let me tell you the difference in an optimist and a pessimist. If you put them in two rooms you can tell the difference. You put the pessimist in a room full of wonderful toys. You put the optimist in a room of horse manure. You come back in two hours and ask the pessimist, 'How are you doing?' He's sitting there with a frown on his face, not playing with anything, and answers, 'Terrible. There's nothing here I like to play with.' Then you go into the room with the optimist. There he is with manure all over his hands and face and all over the room. He's digging with his hands into the manure pile with a smile on his face. When you ask him how he is doing, he says, 'Great! With all of this horse manure, there must be a pony in here somewhere!'"

When you think about terrible health news, particularly if death is coming soon, you certainly have the right to feel you've been placed in a room of manure. Your attitude within that room, however, is your choice. You can choose to live the remainder of your life depressed, saying, "They've taken away all my toys," or you can look for the pony. The truth for the Christian is that the pony is there. God has promised that "in all things" he "works for the good of those who love him" (Rom. 8:28). "In all things" means in a room full of manure, and it means in the face of illness.

How can God bring good out of your misery? The answer will be different for each of us. Some will find a new relationship with God they never would have had without facing that misery. Some will be able to settle old accounts and build relationship bridges that were impossible before. Some will be freed from the expectations of society, finally able to do something they have always wanted to do. Some will be able to just rest for a while after life has pushed them too hard for too long. Some will learn to appreciate a granddaughter's smile when, before facing the illness, that smile had passed in a blur. The good will be different for each person. Physical illness, and all that goes with it, is clearly a room full of manure, but there is a pony there, and you will find it if you keep looking for it. As you face the bad news your doctor has handed you, seek the good, seek God, and with God beside you, you will find the good.

SERIOUS ILLNESS AS A ROSE

One way of searching for the good within the pain of tragic health news is to think of our sufferings as thorns within which roses are hidden. A few years ago Gary Morris performed a song about redeeming love titled "The Love She Found in Me."[1] He sang of a man who felt as though his life was nothing but thorns until a girl came along and found the roses hidden there.

Serious illness, like a rose, is a plant with beautiful blooms and terrible thorns. We often fear these thorns so much that we never pluck the blossom they defend. But some people, like the girl in the song, possess the ability to find the roses within the thorns, the sea beside the sand, and the beautiful rainbow in the cold rain. I have a friend like that. She went through the emotional trauma of her unmarried daughter bearing a child but focused on the wonder and joy that child brought to her life. Later in life, she lost her wealth and was bankrupt, then, in one year's time lost her sister, mother, and father in death. In spite of her pain, she spoke often of how she and her husband had found God in those tragedies. She is a remarkable example of one who sees the good in everything. We all, to some degree, can direct our focus to the good in life, and we can even do that within our illness. If we say there are no roses in our misery, we have given in to the pain of the thorns. There are many roses within the thorns. Let me name a few that may apply to your illness.

The Rose of Uninhibited Relationships

Mary Faith knocked on the door to her sister's apartment, weighed down by the sadness of her sister Cindy's terminal illness. She was surprised by the cheerful response that beckoned her to enter. Walking through the door, she was surprised again to see a smiling face instead of the depression she had expected.

"How are you doing?" asked Mary Faith.

"Great!" answered Cindy.

"What's going on? Why are you happy right now?" asked Mary Faith, a bit incredulously.

"You know my boss, the one who sat and talked with me when I was going through Mom and Dad's divorce? she asked.

"Yeah," answered Mary Faith.

"Now that I'm not worried about my job, I was able to tell him today how much he meant to me as a person, without my being afraid he would think I was looking for a raise. It felt good."

There is a freedom that comes when we realize that many of the social inhibitions around our relationships do not really matter. This becomes crystal clear if you see death in your near future. Not only can you finally be honest with your boss, you can start to say the things that really matter to the people who are important to you. You can tell them things like how much you love them and what is really valuable in your relationship with them. A patient of mine with small cell lung cancer told me one day, "People used to tell me how lucky my wife was to have died suddenly without suffering. I'm the lucky one with my cancer because I'm getting the chance to tell everyone how much they have meant to me."

The Rose of Clarity

So much pressure and information comes flying at us when we struggle through life, seeking to rise to the top, that we often feel overwhelmed yet unable to lighten the load. Often, the discovery that a life-changing illness lies ahead helps dissolve about 90 percent of that information and most of the social pressure. Then, with all that noise gone, we can begin to focus on what really matters—the teenager who needs our time and attention, or the spouse who needs our comfort, or the friend for whom no one else seems to care.

Miriam was a patient of mine with breast cancer. "I never saw the sky before, until I got cancer. I never heard the birds. I never really took the time to love my husband like I should. There was so much other stuff crowding our lives. My life with him is so much better now."

The Rose of Unfettered Mission

Jesus said, "You cannot serve both God and Money" (Matt. 6:24), and yet we spend our lives trying to serve them both. But when we see death ahead, gone is the need to make a good impression, the need to save up for that boat, the need to spend extra time at the office so the boss will be pleased. Whatever time we have left can be spent finally living out the mission that God has created for us. We can tell others about his love and faithfulness without worrying that they may think we are weird. We can give our money to the poor without concern about the loss to our security blanket. We can finally be what God intended and can accomplish the mission that he has sent us into this world to complete. One changed life for him is worth all eternity. Now we can seek those lives that God wants to change.

A young man with brain cancer told me how his cancer had allowed him to minister to his sister. "You know, one good thing that has come out of this cancer is that my sister accepted Christ. She was not a Christian. Recently she developed breast cancer. I think she is going to be fine with the cancer, but when she was talking with me the other day, I was able to ask her the question, 'If you were to die, are you sure that you would spend eternity in heaven?' She would never have accepted that question before, and I would never have asked it. But because of the suffering I have gone through with my cancer, I was able to ask and she was willing to listen. She prayed the sinner's prayer and accepted Christ as her Savior."

Whatever time we have left can be spent living out the mission that God created for us.

THE ROSE OF UNDISCOVERED PLEASURES

Perhaps you've never taken the time to smell any flower and you can smell lots of flowers now. Perhaps you've never sat in a concert and let the music bathe you with relaxing strains; now is a good time. Perhaps you've always wanted to see Mount Rushmore or the Grand Canyon; why not now?

John had one particular dream that was important to him. He was suffering from lung cancer and had little time left to live. He had always wanted a convertible and swore he would not die until he got one. He purchased a Chrysler LeBaron convertible and rode in it one time, having the time of his life. John took advantage of his diminished future responsibilities to find joy for the moment. When serious illness strikes, we have a good excuse to discover some of the good things in this life before we get to the great things in the next life.

God says through Paul, "And we know that in all things God works for the good of those who love him, who have been called according to his purpose" (Rom. 8:28). He's talking about God's ability to reach into a bed of thorns and pull out a rose. Clearly there are many more roses among the thorns of physical suffering than these few we have mentioned. You need to understand, however, that they will not come looking for you to smell their fragrance. When the gloom of bad news is upon you, looking for roses becomes a matter of decision over emotion. You must say, "There are roses here that I will find even though I don't feel like it. I will seek that new relationship. I will focus my life and actions on the truly important. I will seek his mission even within the gloom." Otherwise the rest of your life will be wasted, spent only among the thorns.

We can discover some of the good things in this life before we get to the great things in the next life.

Cultivate a Thankful Heart

One of the best ways to bring joy into our lives is to cultivate a thankful heart. I learned this first in an African village fifteen years ago.

It was another hot day in Sanubi, Nigeria. Earlier, we had felt a hint of breeze inside the sweltering church; we knew it was from God, but the church members felt chilled, so they shut the windows. Becky and I were both drenched in sweat by the time the service ended. But then the service didn't really end. An additional service we had known nothing about began. Our heat exhaustion was soon lost in wonder at the celebration before us. This was the annual Thanksgiving service for Sanubi. I watched in fascination as groups lined up at the back of the church: groups of women, groups of children, groups of men, then groups that were mixed. Some church members joined many different groups before it was over. Each group picked a song of praise or thanksgiving and then sang it as they joyfully clapped their way to the front of the church. Many songs were sung in the Urhobo language. Some were in English. I remember particularly:

What will I render unto my God?
What will I render unto my Savior?
I will give all my life unto Him;
I will give all my life unto Him.

and

I look to my right and see Satan has fallen;
I look to my left and see Satan has fallen;
I look to my front and see Satan has fallen;
I look to my rear and see Satan has fallen;
I have seen, seen the downfall of Satan.
Glory to God, Amen!

As they reached the front of the concrete sanctuary ringing with their joy, the church members placed money on the altar as a gift of gratitude to God for what he had done for them in the past year: farmers for their crops, mothers for their children, children for their parents, and so forth. I, too, was uplifted in joy and gratitude. By the time the service ended, these people had laid five hundred *naira* on the altar. If measured by percentage of yearly salary, in the United States that would have been the equivalent of a 150-member church placing fifty thousand dollars in the offering plate. And these people were the poorest I have ever known. There was more sickness and loss in their lives than any people I have ever met in the world. Yet the joy that came with the Thanksgiving service lifted them above their misery and transformed them from sufferers to servants.

There is no greater way to peace than to have a thankful heart. I have known patients who faced their wounded lives with joy, resting on their gratitude for all they had received during their lives and even during their illness. I have also known people whose lives were filled with bitterness and anger to the end of their days because they had seen nothing for which they felt thankful. There was no difference in the social and physical suffering of these two kinds of people. The only difference was in their attitude toward life.

Betty had advanced ovarian cancer that should have taken her life. She was treated very aggressively with chemotherapy and returned to me ten years later, cured of her malignancy. However, she had developed a blood disorder caused by her treatment that would cause her death within a few years. I have known people who have been very angry and bitter in similar circumstances. Betty simply said, "I am so grateful for the ten years I have been given so far."

Kelsey Zehring was a seven-year-old second grader who loved math and excelled at ballet. Her parents are Christians. She developed a headache one day after school and was dead twelve hours later. I would be angry and bitter if that had been my child, but in the Memphis *Commercial Appeal* Kelsey's father was quoted as saying, "We had a great life. She had seven beautiful years."[2] He was a man with a thankful heart that will keep his bitterness at bay and allow the beauty of his time with Kelsey to survive.

You can have a thankful heart in the midst of great tragedies. Paul knew that. He told us to "give thanks in all circumstances, for this is God's will for you in Christ Jesus" (1 Thess. 5:18). Paul is not saying to be thankful for all circumstances but that in all circumstances we can find something or someone for which we can be thankful. William Barclay, in his commentary on this passage, says, "We must remember that if we face the sun the shadows will fall behind us, but if we turn our backs on the sun, all shadows will be in front."[3]

For what can we really be thankful when the doctor brings terrible news to us or to those we love?

We can be thankful for the good things we had in life. Mrs. Moore was an elderly woman with ovarian cancer. We treated her advanced cancer for over two years. She suffered chronic pain due to the cancer and severe arthritis. One day in my office, after discussing her symptoms, she smiled and said, "God has blessed me with so many good things, Dr. Weir. I don't know why he has been so good to me."

After Mrs. Therell found out that her cancer was progressing and she probably would not have long to live, she told her son, "Don't fret about this. I have had a wonderful year and a half that I was not expected to have in which I got to play with these wonderful grandchildren of mine. I have had time to organize my possessions and give them away. I have had a great time with you. This has been a great year and a half, so I am not going to be depressed, and I don't want you to be either."

These two women were thankful not because they had suffered less than others; but they enjoyed life more because they were thankful.

We can be thankful for the good things remaining in life. My mother-in-law, Nana, lived fully the last years of her life in spite of cancer. One of the greatest joys in her life took place when she was already short of breath from the cancer in her lungs. She traveled with Becky, me, and her grandchildren to Colorado for a week at a family dude ranch. There she was relaxed, surrounded by her beloved daughter and grandchildren and by all of God's glorious mountain scenery to remind her of her Creator and Sustainer. She truly enjoyed that wonderful time, when many would have felt there was nothing left to live for.

We can be thankful for God's presence. In this book I have listed a number of people who have gone through great suffering yet found the presence of God within that suffering. They and many others have said to me, "I am thankful for the suffering because it was there that I found God." Paul said, "I consider everything a loss compared to the surpassing greatness of knowing Christ Jesus my Lord, for whose sake I have lost all things. I consider them rubbish, that I may gain Christ" (Phil. 3:8).

And finally, we can be thankful for victory. Dr. Margarette Sather, a Christian professor of humanities at a respected local university, never voiced despair when she was dying. In fact, as reported in our *Commercial Appeal* newspaper, she planned her death as a celebration. She even planned her last thought, "which will come she hopes in her sleep. She will be cradled in Christ's arms, she says, and be taken away. 'I want to be fit to enter the Presence.' "[4]

Even death is not defeat; it is a victory where death dissolves into perfect life eternal. As Paul says:

> "Death has been swallowed up in victory."
> "Where, O death, is your victory?

> Where, O death, is your sting?"
>
> The sting of death is sin, and the power of sin is the law. But thanks be to God! He gives us victory through our Lord Jesus Christ.
>
> —1 CORINTHIANS 15:54–57

You can keep a thankful heart when serious illness strikes. It is one clear way to keep your happiness alive.

TWELVE

Choose to Manage Your Emotions

Jesus served the Last Supper and watched Judas go out to betray him. He pronounced his imminent death to his disciples and warned of Peter's upcoming denial. They all, except Judas, left the Upper Room together and walked to a private olive garden, where they stopped, and Jesus went on alone. Jesus fell to his knees and pleaded to avoid his own suffering and death. His heart was filled with sadness and turmoil. Nevertheless, he understood that his Father's will was through a way of great sadness, and he accepted that will, rose from his knees, and went on with his life in the midst of the sadness (Matt. 26:36–46).

All my life I've heard people say they were confident they were within the will of God because of the peace and joy they felt. I came to believe that I, too, could identify how close I was to God's plan by the degree of peace and joy I was experiencing. Then, when God called Becky and me to take our family to Nigeria, I was left with a dilemma.

I really felt no joy at the thought of going. God had clearly spoken to us to go, but I had no peace about it. I wanted to enter foreign missions with a desire to heal the suffering and carry God's Word to people I loved, but I had never known a Nigerian. My mind and God's direction were very clear, but my heart lagged far behind. God pulled me to Nigeria while my emotions were pulling elsewhere. It was after I arrived in Nigeria that I fell in love with the Nigerian people and the work there. I expect I will never find work that is as satisfying to me as those two years in Eku, Nigeria. It was after I began the work that the joy and peace came. I remember one morning specifically in the dark early African hours when I sat at my kitchen table, spending my time with the Father before starting hospital rounds. At that moment in an emotional slump, I was unhappy with my early morning hours, unhappy with my living conditions, saddened by my wife's loneliness, and wishing I were back in Memphis again. At that table before the sun rose over the palm trees, God made it very clear to me that I was where he wanted me to be. With that clear assurance, all those depressing emotions that filled my heart no longer mattered. God's plan and God's presence were more important than my feeling happy, and I could walk in his will in spite of the absence of joy and peace for a while. It was a liberating moment in my life. I was freed from the wild fluctuations in my emotions; I did not have to do what they said anymore.

Matthew 26:36–44 reminds us that Jesus was alone in the Garden of Gethsemane prior to his death and was terribly sad; he was afraid; he cried for God to change his mind. But Jesus continued to follow God's will through it all.

It can be very difficult to shake the gloom and sadness that comes with the realization of serious illness. We can make the mistake of letting that emotional depression make us feel that we are separated from God. We may even feel guilty that we cannot feel the peace and joy that others have demonstrated in their suffering. When I left Nigeria, my emotions pulled me to stay there, just as they had earlier pulled me to remain in Memphis. In both situations, God's presence and will were greater than my emotions. It's great to feel joy and peace. I believe that those who walk with God will experience far more joy and peace in their lives than those who do not follow God. But the presence of these emotions is not a guarantee of God's presence, plan, or love for us; just as their absence is not indicative of his absence or displeasure. As long as we live in this world, we need to feel free to experience sadness yet still cling to his hand. We need to accept our tears while still walking in his footsteps. Eventually the joy and peace we experience will be far beyond anything we have ever known, and it will be continual and everlasting. But while we are here in this world, let us tolerate and express our emotions without allowing them to rule our lives.

ANGER

One of the emotions that comes naturally when facing a serious health problem is anger. Anger is normal, but it can drain the joy from the rest of our lives.

As long as we live in this world, we need to feel free to experience sadness, yet still cling to his hand.

Martha's family flew her in from Pensacola to let her die at home with her son in Memphis. She was only forty-seven and stared into space, unable to speak. She had been diagnosed with a brain tumor. Three weeks before she had been walking, talking, and normal. It seemed to me that something was not quite right with her diagnosis. She had deteriorated too rapidly. Even though she had come to die, I suggested that perhaps we should be certain about the pathology, and I sent for the slides from Pensacola.

By the next day, however, the neurological signs were devastating. Her pupils were dilated, and she was posturing in a way that told me her brain was beyond recovery. I stood in the hall with her son and told him that whatever the diagnosis, she would not recover. I told him that the family was in charge, but if she were my mother, I would let her die without putting her on a ventilator and without putting her through a lot of difficult tests. I thought he understood, and I detected no unusual emotional energy. When I reached the office, however, the son and his sister had both called, boiling mad. They accused me of wanting to let their mother die. They wanted another doctor and two other opinions. Their anger was intense.

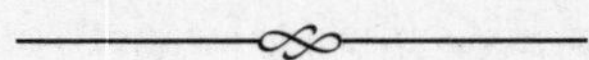

Anger is a part of facing serious illness, whether it is our own illness or that of someone we love. It boils up within us. We may not want it there or even know what it is, but we can't prevent it. What can we do with the anger that grips us when the doctor brings us bad news?

Causes of Anger

I know of four causes of anger, though psychologists probably can cite many more.

1. Anger is a response to pain. When Bowen accidentally rolls over my hand with his roller skates, my immediate response is anger. I still love him, but the pain in my hand makes me angry. The doctor's bad news brings the fear and reality of both physical and emotional pain, so anger often follows.

2. Anger is a response to loss of personal rights. Bessie is a composite of many young parents I have known who discovered they had incurable cancer. "It's not fair," she said. "My daughter is only eight years old. I should get to see her play soccer and go out on her first date. She needs me; I'm her mother." It is normal to be angry when an illness threatens to take away our right to continue the life we have started.

3. Anger is a response to loss of personal control. Matthew was a top executive. Now he had cancer and an injury to his spine. His business partners were in his hospital room trying to transfer some of his responsibilities over to other corporate workers. Matthew was in pain but would not show it. He felt terrible, but he was clean shaven and had his hair styled. He had decided he would not show his pain or weakness. He was still in charge.

As his associate leaned over the bed to review a particular line on one contract, a terrible odor rose in the room, and Matthew realized that his bowels had emptied without warning. His face turned red, but he remained composed. Through lips that barely moved, he ordered, "Everyone leave the room!" When the room emptied, his anger turned to tears.

When serious illness overtakes us, it often strips from us our control over our own lives—physically, emotionally, and financially. Things happen to us that we cannot stop, and we grow angry.

4. Anger is a response to dreams denied. I returned from the mission field due to health problems within my family. Except for short-term mission work, we never went back. It took me seven years to finally give up the dream of returning to Africa. I can remember that morning clearly. With the knowledge that my dream had died, I began running, and with the energy born of anger, I did not stop until I had run seven miles and collapsed in total physical and spiritual exhaustion. Just so, when a devastating health problem comes into view, our dreams for the future may come crashing down and leave us angry at the dream denied.

Anger is an inevitable part of facing serious illness, and many problems come with anger. One is that anger never hurts the illness we are facing; instead it usually misses the mark and hits innocent bystanders. We may even aim our anger at God, who is our one hope in passing through death to life. Our anger may strike our families, whom we ought to be showering with love. Anger most often boomerangs and comes back to strike us with guilt, depression, and smoldering resentment. Rather than helping us in our new difficulties, it adds huge and painful burdens and separates us from God and those we love.

Removing Anger

If anger is your enemy, how do you remove it so you do not feel its sting? I learned five principles from Dr. David Allen, a brilliant and compassionate Christian psychologist, at a retreat for Christian physicians when I most needed them in my own life.

1. Recognize the anger. It may be that as you look ahead toward a serious illness, you may feel terrible emotionally and not know why. You need to investigate your emotions and see if there is anger in your life. You need to do this prayerfully, with God's help. Psalm 139 speaks to this need:

> Search me, O God, and know my heart;
> test me and know my anxious thoughts.
> See if there is any offensive way in me,
> and lead me in the way everlasting.
>
> —PSALM 139:23–24

2. Rationalize the anger. It may be that you have identified the anger but don't understand why it is there or why it is pointed in a given direction. Often the manifestation and direction of our anger do not make sense.

I worked closely with Sue, a nurse whom I respect very much. Her mother became sick with cancer and died. Sometime after her mother's death, Sue told my office nurse that she hated her mother's doctor. She hated him because her mother had died in pain, and her doctor had refused to help her. I sat down with Sue and worked out the full story. Her mother's doctor was not on call the weekend she died. Sue's mother had been hurting, so she contacted the covering physician, who provided pain medicine. The mother and her family never called back to tell the doctor that the medicine was inadequate, and the mother died in pain. The doctor was unaware of her mother's pain, and her pain was managed appropriately according to the information provided. As Sue worked through the facts, her anger gradually diminished.

It is important to make your anger rational, to know the real cause and to whom it really should be directed, and to know the most appropriate action that should result from that anger. Sometimes the focus of the anger needs to be redirected from a person to the illness itself, and the appropriate action is to grieve in the arms of God.

3. Relinquish the rights. Many times a patient will tell me, "I did everything God wanted. I don't deserve this. It is my right to live because I have been good," or "How can God do this to my children? They are innocent; they have a right not to live without their mother." Much of anger comes from being robbed of such personal rights.

When a Libyan henchman held a machete over the head of missionary Ralph Bethea and shouted, "Are you ready to die, Christian?" Ralph replied, "I can't die, sir; I am already dead." This young missionary understood the words of the apostle Paul, "For you died, and your life is now hidden with Christ in God" (Col. 3:3). Ralph Bethea had long before surrendered the rights to his life and handed them to God.

Jamie Boelter tells of the ordeal she went through in accepting the illness of her husband, Rick. "I told God I wanted his will, but I could not give him my husband. One day I was reading the Bible and praying for Rick when the Scripture hit me right between the eyes and tore into my heart. I knew what I must do. Face down on the floor, I gave my husband to God, whatever his will." It was then that God was able to work a great thing in Rick's and Jamie's lives. Our lives are secure only if we transfer them from our own hands to the hands of God. We cannot be angry at the taking of our life if we have already given it to God to do with what he wills. It is the same with our children but even harder. At some time we must release our children to God, for they are his in the first place. Even if we are forced to be separated from them for a while by death, we have already given them to the Father, whom we trust to care for them. When we relinquish our rights and hand them to God, sickness and death cannot steal them from us.

4. Relate the anger. Perhaps before you understood the anger that comes from facing your illness, that anger had already struck out and injured someone you love. Once you have discovered that anger, made it rational, and relinquished the right that led to the pain, you need to share your feelings of anger with God, with those you love, and specifically with anyone who might have been hurt by that anger.

I have already told you the story of our patient with breast cancer who came each week to receive her chemotherapy in a visibly angry mood. My nurse began to pry gently week by week to find the source of her anger. We assumed it was because of her illness, but one day the patient told my nurse of a broken relationship with her sister that had developed into an angry resentment over the years. My nurse encouraged her to contact her sister and attempt to make amends. At her next visit, the patient came in visibly peaceful for the first time. She had visited her sister that week and laid down her anger. She was happier than she had been in years in spite of the cancer she faced. When you lay down your anger, healing can occur between you, God, and your loved ones. Then the rest of your life can be open to real intimacy rather than be walled off and isolated by the barrier of resentment and hurt.

5. *Release the anger.* A young patient of mine who loves the Lord has been through terrible treatments for a lymphoma around his brain. He is suing his ophthalmologist, who had noted an abnormality months before his diagnosis was made but did not follow up on it to find the lymphoma. The lawsuit is not based on a desire for money but comes out of anger for the young man's suffering. "He's got to pay for what he has done to me. We can't let him do this to anyone else." The truth is, the anger possibly will result in much-needed money but will also add frustration, anxiety, and further anger to a life that is most in need of peace.

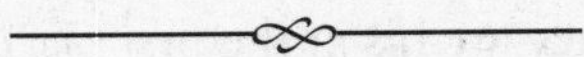

God will not steal our anger from us if we choose to wrap our hearts in it. But if we release our anger and lay it at his feet, he will bear it for us and give us instead a new heart and a steadfast spirit to face the trials ahead.

It's Okay to Cry

A word of caution: letting go of our anger and dealing with our emotions does not mean forsaking all emotions. Letting go of anger does not mean dropping the emotional content of our lives and living with artificial happiness. Our emotions are God-given, and we should not seek to live the rest of our lives numb from feeling in order to avoid the pain.

A young Christian puppeteer and play therapist at our Memphis children's hospital told us this story at a gathering of Christian medical and dental students:

Jason and Erica were patients at the hospital and shared a ward. When the phlebotomist came to draw their blood for laboratory tests, both were frightened, but they reacted differently to the threat. Jason was nine and, as a boy that age, proving his courage was everything. When the phlebotomist asked for his arm, he held it out rigid, stared into a corner, and took the pain like a man. You could see his chest stick out in pride after the bloodletting had confirmed his toughness.

Our emotions are God-given; we should not seek to live numb from feeling in order to avoid the pain.

Erica was only six and showed her terror. She could not voluntarily hold out her arm, and even when they held it still for her, she squirmed and screamed and cried with gusto. After she was finished, Jason looked at her with prideful contempt.

The nurse came to Jason with a Popsicle and held it out to him, "This Popsicle's for you, Jason, because you were so brave and cooperative, and you didn't cry." Jason accepted the Popsicle with a grin, then cut his eyes toward Erica, whose head was tucked down in embarrassment. The nurse then held out another Popsicle, "Erica, you get a Popsicle too because it hurt you so bad." Erica's head rose, and she was beaming as she took it.

By this time, the phlebotomist had reached the ward next door, and the scream of a child rang out down the hospital corridor. Jason continued to enjoy his Popsicle in spite of the noise. Erica, however, slipped out of bed and walked down the hall to the room where the current needle victim was suffering. She stood at the door until the phlebotomist left, then walked over to the crying girl and handed her the Popsicle she had received and said, "It's okay. I cried too."

It is okay to cry when faced with suffering and death. David had a child with Bathsheba. One day the child became ill and appeared to be dying. "David pleaded with God for the child. He fasted and went into his house and spent the nights lying on the ground. The elders of his household stood beside him to get him up from the ground, but he refused, and he would not eat any food with them" (2 Sam. 12:16–17). For seven days David cried his eyes and heart out for the child he loved. On the seventh day,

> David noticed that his servants were whispering among themselves and he realized the child was dead. "Is the child dead?" he asked.
>
> "Yes," they replied, "he is dead."
>
> David got up from the ground. After he had washed, put on lotions and changed his clothes, he went into the house of the Lord and worshiped. Then he went to his own house, and at his request they served him food, and he ate.
>
> His servants asked him, "Why are you acting this way? While the child was alive, you fasted and wept, but now that the child is dead, you get up and eat!"
>
> He answered, "While the child was still alive, I fasted and wept. I thought, 'Who knows? The Lord may be gracious to me and let the child live.' But now that he is dead, why should I fast? Can I bring him back again? I will go to him, but he will not return to me."
>
> —2 Samuel 12:19–23

David cried and pleaded for a time, but when he realized his wishes were not to come true, he turned to God in trust and worshiped him.

Like David, Jesus cried for the suffering ahead. As he faced death on the Cross, he cried and in anguish sweated drops like blood. Jesus says to us as we contemplate suffering or death, "It's okay. I cried too." Crying in our pain is real. It is human and honest and blessed by God. But after Jesus had cried and prayed for a time, he said, "My Father, if it is not possible for this cup to be taken away unless I drink it, may your will be done" (Matt. 26:42). Then he rose from his tears and his prayers, gathered his disciples, and faced his death while trusting in his Father.

You cannot face your suffering without the human anguish that comes with it, and God says it is okay to cry. David cried and Jesus cried. When little Erica cried, she still got a Popsicle, and when we cry, God still holds out his loving arms. He will not draw them back because you show your suffering. Those arms are there to carry you through. After a while, however, the tears should diminish, not because your pain is less, but because your trust is more.

THIRTEEN

Choose to Pursue Peace

David was a great man, but he was an imperfect man, as we all are. He could not control his desire for Bathsheba, and he often failed as a father. Absalom was the son David loved the most, yet Absalom did not love him. The time came when Absalom successfully revolted against the father who loved him. David fled from Jerusalem, and Absalom entered the palace to sleep with David's wives (see 2 Sam. 15–16). Here we see David the king become David the refugee. The one who had everything that anyone could wish for in life, lost it all and faced probable death. Here also we can gain lessons of strength for those who face loss or death, whatever the cause.

The depth of chapters 15 and 16 of 2 Samuel was first revealed to me by Dr. David Allen when I was going through a time of loss in my life, at the same retreat mentioned earlier. Walk now a few minutes with me and David the king and see if his steps to peace can be your own.

Face the Problem

The first step David took when told of his son's rebellion and advance on the palace was to face the problem: "A messenger came and told

David, 'The hearts of the men of Israel are with Absalom.' Then David said to his officials who were with him in Jerusalem, 'Come! We must flee, or none of us will escape from Absalom. We must leave immediately, or he will move quickly to overtake us and bring ruin upon us and put the city to the sword'" (2 Sam. 15:13–14).

One of the easiest ways mentally to escape a tragedy is to deny its existence. I remember particularly a man in his fifties who had advanced lung cancer with a large mass in his chest and palpable masses of tumor at the base of his neck. In spite of the biopsies, bronchoscopy, and X rays, he still denied he had cancer. He died denying his sickness. Many other patients accept the truth of their diagnosis, but denial comes when they refuse to believe that their problem cannot be fixed. They spend the rest of their lives moving from one improbable cure to the next, losing the time they could have spent squeezing value out of the life they had left. Other patients I have known use their faith as a mechanism for denial. "I have faith that God has healed me." Sometimes God does heal. But in truth, most of the time those who claim divine healing have *hope that faith will heal them, not faith that God will heal them.* All Christians with faith someday pass through the gate of death into the arms of God, and usually it comes to pass near the time that science has predicted. Most of the time, in health issues, scientific truth is God's truth as well.

There are other patients who are not so drastic in their denial. Instead of claiming to be healed, they choose not to discuss their disease after the diagnosis is announced. They then relegate all further discussions to family members, particularly discussions about the expected duration of their lives. Sometimes the children take on the role of denial for their parents. I am very often exasperated when I approach the room of a new cancer patient in his sixties or seventies and find the door blockaded by his grown children. They demand that I not tell their parent of the cancer diagnosis or of the truth regarding his life expectancy. I then enter the room and find a perfectly competent patient who needs to understand his diagnosis in order to make decisions regarding treatment and in order to make plans for the life that does remain.

I have also known remarkable people like Dr. Margarette Sather, the professor I mentioned earlier, who (as reported in a local newspaper, the *Commercial Appeal*) announced to her colleagues, "I have cancer, and I will die soon. Talk to me about it. I am a Christian, and I am not afraid."[1] Denial is a tool that may temporarily and artificially soothe the fear of approaching suffering or death, but it interferes with appropriate decision-making for the life remaining and builds a wall of silence between patients and families at a time when intimacy and communication become more important than ever before.

David the king could have denied Absalom's threat and said, "It is not true. You are talking about my son. He would never kill his father. Even if it is true, once he sees me, he will change his mind." If David had done that, then he, like my lung cancer patient, would have died in denial. When serious illness is near, we must face the problem and make appropriate decisions based on the truth.

FEEL THE PAIN

David did not face his tragedy stoically or mechanically. He accepted his loss and probable death as fact, and he felt the pain. "But David continued up the Mount of Olives, weeping as he went; his head was covered and he was barefoot" (2 Sam. 15:30). It is okay to cry for a while. It is okay to feel the pain, at times. God made us creatures who long to hold on to life, so letting go hurts.

> *Feel the pain and cry for a while, but then tame it. Sorrow can grow into a monster that destroys the happiness of your remaining days.*

As we said earlier, even our Master felt the pain. "They went to a place called Gethsemane, and Jesus said to his disciples, 'Sit here while I pray.' He took Peter, James and John along with him, and he began to be deeply distressed and troubled. 'My soul is overwhelmed with sorrow to the point of death,' he said to them" (Mark 14:32–34). Like Jesus, it is appropriate for you to feel deeply the sorrow that comes with your illness. You must feel the pain and cry for a while, but then you must tame it. Sorrow uncontrolled can grow into a monster that destroys the happiness of your remaining days. Sorrow uncontrolled leads to anger, which must be released if you are to find peace.

Recognize God's Providence

David faced the problem, felt the pain, and recognized God's providence. We have read the passage that tells of King David as he was climbing the hills out of Jerusalem. Zadok the priest followed him with the ark of the covenant, representing the presence of God. Rather than presuming God would choose his side in the conflict, David said to Zadok, "Take the ark of God back into the city. If I find favor in the LORD's eyes, he will bring me back. . . . But if he says, 'I am not pleased with you,' then I am ready; let him do whatever seems good to him" (2 Sam. 15:25–26). Centuries before David, that man of God, Job, in all of his misery, put it this way: "Though he slay me, yet will I trust in him" (Job 13:15 KJV).

Richard was one of my favorite patients. He was over eighty years old and had severe anemia, heart disease, and cirrhosis. He knew he probably would not live on earth much longer. He was a neat old guy who finally had received his college degree at sixty years of age and spent his spare time tutoring football players for free. Once I asked him how he was coping. He smiled as he answered, "I'm in good hands; I'm in the Lord's hands. I've got the best doctors of anywhere in the world. If things don't work out, I know where I'm going, so how can I be blue?" Richard released his remaining days into God's loving care and lived in peace until he died.

One way of denying God's providence is by demanding answers to questions that will not be answered on this side of eternity. One such rarely answered question is "Why?" All the theologians in the world cannot answer this question satisfactorily, yet when we see our suffering ahead, we instinctively ask it.

One of my Christian friends, a talented editor, several years ago decided to observe Lent by giving up the question "Why?" She says of that experience, "I've not yet resumed the practice of asking it and consider that to be one of the smallest, most liberating things I've ever done!"

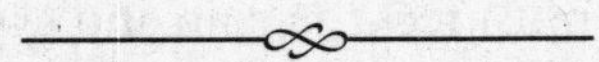

I am told that in the church that covers the spot of the Garden of Gethsemane where Jesus felt such intense sorrow, there is a sign requesting silence. It reads, "Please, no explanations in church." Jesus received no explanations as to why he must die when he wept in the garden, but he laid his death in the hands of God. We will receive no satisfactory explanation for our own suffering or the suffering of those we love on this side of death, so let us ask the question once, because it demands to come out of us; then let it go and settle into the comfort of God's hands.

RETURN TO ACTION

David faced the problem, felt the pain, and recognized God's providence. Then when his march to escape was over, he returned to action. Men had gathered under David from throughout the countryside. He could now give up with his own son against him, or he could return to the battles of life and live out God's purpose for him in this world. "David mustered the men who were with him and appointed over them commanders of thousands and commanders of hundreds. David sent the troops out" (2 Sam. 18:1–2). In spite of the heartache, loss, and probable death ahead, David passed through the sorrow and entered life again.

I have a remarkable young patient who came to me one year ago with a cancer that had popped up in various parts of her body and was incurable from the day we met. Rather than stopping work, collecting disability, and dropping out of life, she bought a wig, continued to date actively, and hardly missed a step in life in spite of her cancer, its treatment, or the specter of her death. Another middle-aged patient of mine still works regularly and rarely complains even though she has breast cancer and chronic back pain and requires portable oxygen to breathe. I don't know if they will live longer because of their determination, but I know that their ability to enjoy life, to squeeze the goodness out of life, is markedly enhanced by their attitude.

There are many difficulties ahead in your diagnosis as well, but there is life between diagnosis and death. We can either sit in a corner and wait until the end or live out the life we were given and accomplish fully the intention for which we were sent. Face the problem, feel the pain for a while, recognize God's providence, and get back into the living of life. These actions are the scissors that God has placed in your hands to cut the bands of anguish from around your heart and give you peace.

I have mentioned the story of Murray Alexander, whose life with cancer had brought him so close to God that he would rather keep the cancer than lose that relationship. He knew that seeking the presence of God was the greatest need in the midst of his suffering. Soon after he learned that his cancer was in remission, he wrote an open letter to his family.

> Dear Family,
>
> The longer you live, the more you will realize that life is not always fair. You will learn that bad things do happen to good people. I want to tell you a true story that, I hope, can help you through some of these hard times.
>
> In January of 1993, I was in my sixty-seventh year. Earlier, I had retired after farming the home place for over forty years and was feeling good while enjoying the freedom that retirement gave me.
>
> About this time, I began to look around and realized that some bad physical things were happening to folks my age and that this could happen to me. The main thing that I feared was getting cancer. I wasn't afraid of dying—I had gotten that settled with the Lord long ago—but I did fear the dying process. I didn't want to suffer like that, so in my quiet time I began to pray that I be spared from this. Gradually the prayer changed to a request that, if it did happen, He would help me to handle it right—that I would not be an embarrassment to Him by the way I reacted—that He would help me be the same type of person when things got tough that I had professed to be when things were going my way.
>
> Six months later I was found to have a mass in my kidney, and the most wonderful things began to happen in my life. This is what I want to pass on to you all because there will be a time when you will desperately need it.

When I heard the doctor tell Nanny that "here's the problem, he has a mass," it was like a bright light suddenly coming on in a dark room. I thought, "Well, here it is. This is what God has been preparing me for all this time—it's in His hands and He will work it out somehow." At this moment the words of Jesus to His disciples in John 14:27 went through my mind when He told them, "Peace I give you—let not your heart be troubled, neither let it be afraid." Just then, the most profound sense of His peace covered me like a blanket, and I was not afraid. I don't mean that I handled the fear or that I conquered the fear—I mean that there was no fear. There was nothing that I did, no show of courage—it was a gift.

Well, as things sometimes do, it got worse. Four months later the renal cell cancer had spread to my liver, and I was only given from three months to a year to live. I was also given less than a 10 percent chance of even responding to the best known treatment. A second opinion confirmed this. The future looked grim, but that wonderful sense of God's peace remained. I felt like a spectator to an event, not as one who was participating. Each day was a whole new life, and was it ever appreciated.

I began treatment in Memphis under a wonderful oncologist. The only drug that might help was a relatively new one called Interleukin 2, which is completely opposite from the chemo drugs. It jump starts and speeds up the disease-fighting antibodies that we all produce instead of just killing both good and bad cells. This seemed to be helping some, but then I became allergic and all treatment stopped. After this, there was only prayer, and there must have been thousands of these from all sorts of people. The strange thing was that I never felt comfortable praying for healing myself. It wasn't that I doubted that God could or would heal but rather that I wanted the best and knew that I didn't have the wisdom and foresight to really know what would ultimately be the best. I did ask that if things got really rough, He would hold my hand.

I wish I had the words to describe to you how I felt those next months. I really believed that, medically and mathematically, I didn't have long to live, but there was no feeling of giving up or of despair. Each day was wonderful, a new gift. My family, my friends, my church became even more dear. My marriage, which had always been good, became better and better. We laughed a lot—we hugged a lot. Even the normal irritations that crop up in every home were pushed aside with a laugh, because on a scale of zero to ten, they were now worth less than zero. Your Nanny was a rock. She took care of me, but she also let me live without smothering me. I know that she was fearful and surely cried sometimes, but not around me. The entire period was the most wonderful time in my life, and the words from John kept going through my mind day and night—thousands of times—and the peace was real and alive, not just words in a book.

Even though surgery is not the norm with renal cell cancer, the doctors finally decided to try to buy some time by performing a new experimental freezing procedure on the tumors. The doctor who developed this practice came to Memphis from New Jersey to perform the procedure as a teaching session at U.T. Medical.

The morning of the surgery, Nanny came rushing into the room and said, "You won't believe what the ONE verse of Scripture is in our devotional for today—John 14:27." Can you even imagine the mathematical probabilities of that one verse being there on the very day I was going into major-major surgery? I have never heard God's audible voice, but I very definitely felt His actual presence at that moment. It couldn't have been any more real if it had arrived by mail. I didn't know if I was going to live or die, but I did know that whatever happened, it was going to be alright. I doubt if they had ever rolled a more laid-back surgery patient into that room as I was on that day.

> The doctors had three surprises waiting for them. There were more tumors than they had thought; they were much larger than the scans had indicated (one almost as big as my fist); and the surgeon said, "Those are the deadest looking tumors I have ever seen." The tests later confirmed that this was so. When Nanny tried to thank the doctor, he quickly told her, "Don't thank me, the Lord healed that man." I think that doctor was right on target. I think that I was healed, at least for the time being, and am extremely thankful. I did want to live, but by far, the most wonderful thing that happened to me through all of this is what I want to share with you. This is the fact that I have been shown that when God offers us His peace, He's not just talking. This peace is for real and is available to us if we just give in and accept it. I learned that if we can find this peace, nothing else really matters, but if we don't find that peace then things can't get good enough to keep us satisfied. . . .
>
> —MURRAY ALEXANDER[2]

Not only must we trust our God, we must also seek him desperately in the midst of our suffering. Once we are in his presence, we know that he is able to do all things and that all he does is motivated by his love for us. More than that, in his arms we feel safe, and we know that all is well.

FOURTEEN

Choose to Let Others Help

The apostle Paul had been to Athens, trying to explain to Greek Gentiles the meaning of Christ's coming into the world. A few had been convinced, but many more had laughed at him. He left there for Corinth, where Aphrodite was queen and most people were satisfied with life. He walked into this city, after being considered of little importance in Athens, and tried again. He began by teaching in the synagogues, but the Jews didn't buy it; they became abusive.

Fed up with all that the Jews had done to him, filled with self-pity, fatigue, and anger, Paul declared, "I've had all that I can stand. I'm through with you. I'll go to the Gentiles only." He moved next door from the synagogue and was able to bring a few Gentiles to Christ, but he remained discouraged.

Paul, a Jew of Jews, was no longer able to witness to the people he loved most. He was now witnessing to the Gentiles, whom he had grown up hating. Paul had given all that he could for the Lord, was bone tired, and saw little hope for success. In the midst of Paul's discouragement, God came to Paul in a vision and offered great words of comfort and vision: "Do not be afraid; keep on speaking, do not be silent. For I am with you, and no one is going to attack and harm you, because I have many people in this city" (Acts 18:9–10).

When the doctor hands us bad news, we very often feel alone and in that aloneness, like Paul, become discouraged. I believe we can hear the words spoken to Paul and take them as words for us and learn to live on with strength. Here is what God said:

"Do Not Be Afraid"

How many times has God in his Word told us not to be afraid? We need to read and remember each of these passages. We need to return to them over and over when fear squeezes the joy out of our lives:

> Then he got into the boat and his disciples followed him. Without warning, a furious storm came up on the lake, so that the waves swept over the boat. But Jesus was sleeping. The disciples went and woke him, saying, "Lord, save us! We're going to drown!"
>
> He replied, "You of little faith, why are you so afraid?" Then he got up and rebuked the winds and the waves, and it was completely calm.
>
> The men were amazed and asked, "What kind of man is this? Even the winds and waves obey him!"
>
> —Matthew 8:23–27

> Are not two sparrows sold for a penny? Yet not one of them will fall to the ground apart from the will of your Father. And even the very hairs of your head are all numbered. So don't be afraid; you are worth more than many sparrows.
>
> —Matthew 10:29–31

> While Jesus was still speaking, some men came from the house of Jairus, the synagogue ruler. "Your daughter is dead," they said. "Why bother the teacher any more?"
>
> Ignoring what they said, Jesus told the synagogue ruler, "Don't be afraid; just believe."
>
> —Mark 5:35–36

> Peace I leave with you; my peace I give you. I do not give to you as the world gives. Do not let your hearts be troubled and do not be afraid.
>
> —JOHN 14:27

> Even though I walk
> through the valley of the shadow of death,
> I will fear no evil,
> for you are with me.
>
> —PSALM 23:4

> The Lord is my light and my salvation—
> whom shall I fear?
> The Lord is the stronghold of my life—
> of whom shall I be afraid?
>
> —PSALM 27:1

> He who dwells in the shelter of the Most High
> will rest in the shadow of the Almighty.
> I will say of the Lord, "He is my refuge and my fortress,
> my God, in whom I trust."
> He will cover you with his feathers,
> and under his wings you will find refuge. . . .
> You will not fear the terror of night.
>
> —PSALM 91:1–2, 4–5

The future always holds much about which we can be afraid. The storms of life may be thrashing our boat, so we are tossed about with no control; we are about to go under. We may feel as helpless as a sparrow falling from the sky with no one to catch us. Our bodies may no longer be able to run alongside our dreams. In the midst of these fears, our Father, through his Word, cries out to us, "I can calm the sea; I know you are falling. Don't be afraid; just believe. I am with you, and my peace I leave with you. I am your light. I am your salvation. I am your strength. I will cover you with my feathers, and the night will not threaten you." God said to Paul in his discouragement, "Do not be afraid." He speaks the same to you over and over, and he tells you that you do not have to face your fear alone.

"I AM WITH YOU"

The disciples had heard this before as Jesus was leaving them. Now Paul needed to hear this as he felt alone and discouraged. You need to hear this as you face a difficult life ahead. As you continue to work and live and walk a difficult road, God is with you. His power is with you; His peace is with you. His person is with you. You walk not alone.

"NO ONE WILL HARM YOU"

Some day Paul, too, would die. But no one would harm him until God had completed Paul's work on this earth. Paul was certain about this, "Being confident of this, that he who began a good work in you will carry it on to completion until the day of Christ Jesus" (Phil. 1:6). We do have God's protection until he is ready to take us home. As long as our task is unfinished, no one will harm us, and even death can only brush us gently one day, as we pass through to continue our walk with God.

A young woman named Renee taught me this confidence. She had breast cancer and not long to live. After visiting her room one day, I got up to leave and wished her well. Renee smiled and responded, "I'm going to be fine. Either the medicine will work and God will heal me here, or it won't work and God will heal me in heaven." With that understanding and God at her side, nothing could really harm Renee, just as nothing can really harm any of us.

"I HAVE MANY PEOPLE IN THE CITY"

God's support for you in your trouble is somewhat like an Oreo cookie. The cream in the middle is "No one will harm you." On top of that central truth is God himself, "I am with you." Then underneath, God grants you further support with the other side of the Oreo: "I have many people in the city."

When Paul was discouraged and felt alone, God told him, "You are not alone. I am with you, and there are people with you as well. Look around. My people in this city are ready to help you, and there are other people here who need to be brought to me. You are not in this alone."

When you look toward a future of dreams broken by the doctor's bad news, you can focus on the crisis, the fear, and the discouragement, or you can focus on God and focus on people. There are people around you to help you, people through whom God's power flows. There are people around you whom you can still serve. There are people whom you can still comfort. There are people who still need the Lord and need you to introduce them to him. God tells us to cease dwelling on ourselves. If you need help, God sends people to give it. If you feel your usefulness is over, you are wrong; there are people still waiting for you to serve.

Elijah the prophet fled Jezebel and wept at Mount Horeb. Discouraged and alone, he felt as Paul would many years later, and perhaps as you do today. Elijah said, "I am the only one left." But God said, "'Yet I reserve seven thousand in Israel—all whose knees have not bowed down to Baal and all whose mouths have not kissed him.' So Elijah went from there and found Elisha son of Shaphat. He was plowing with twelve yoke of oxen, and he himself was driving the twelfth pair. Elijah went up to him and threw his cloak around him" (1 Kings 19:18–19).

If you feel your usefulness is over, you are wrong; there are people still waiting for you to serve.

Elijah thought he was alone and had to face his trouble and despair with no human hands to hold on to. But God said, "You are blind, man. I've got seven thousand others like you in Israel who trust me and are there for you." Elijah found Elisha, and they were together until Elijah was carried to heaven.

Jade's husband left her with two teenagers and a breast cancer that would take her life in less than a year. No one felt more alone than Jade. And then her family, church, and friends gathered around her. Someone paid the counseling fees for her teenage daughter. Transportation for her medical appointments and meals were arranged. Friends were there to hold her and talk to her. Jade was not alone.

Sometimes in your discouragement you may feel, like Paul and Elijah, that you are all alone. No one knows or understands or is able to really help. But God knows, God understands, and God created us not as individuals but as a community of faith. When Christ left this earth, he left the church—Christians holding each other up and fighting on together in his name until the task is done and his kingdom comes. If you face life alone, you will fail. If you face your illness alone, you will fail. You need someone with whom to pray, to fight, and to rest. Find a friend. Find the community of faith. Open up and allow them to do what God has called them to do. Never again walk this life alone.

This idea of community is critical. Much of our lives we feel like we can take on the world. And then there are times we realize that, on our own, we are not enough.

If you face life and your illness alone, you will fail. Find a friend. Never again walk this life alone.

One of my fond memories is of Boy Scout camp in the eighth grade. I was the patrol leader of the Fox Patrol, and we were part of a great Jamboree with competition between scout troops from all over the South. We had a number of skills like fire-starting and compass-navigating in which individuals of expert skill in our patrol could score points for us. I remember that Jack LeBlanc and I set the record for the Jamboree in fire-starting with flint and cotton gauze. I was a proud adolescent.

I particularly remember one event that required more than the expert individual. I can still envision the ten-foot wooden wall that was erected for our whole patrol to get over. Fat, thin, tall, short, weak, and strong had to get over that wall. We put our strongest guy on the bottom to boost those ahead of him. That was not me. Someone started the time clock, and we all ran to the wall. The strong guy at the base cupped his hands for the others to step in and then boosted them up until they could grasp the top ledge to pull themselves over. Our big boy got pretty tired lifting the rest of us, but that was not our patrol's greatest difficulty. When the strong guy had boosted the last man to the top, he was left by himself, alone in the dirt, with the wall too high to climb. The only way we got our last man over the wall was for the last two guys he boosted to stay at the top, grab his arms as he jumped, then pull him over with us.

Perhaps you have always been the one to boost others over the high walls of life. Perhaps now, with the doctor's bad news, you find yourself standing in the dirt with a wall too high for you to climb. The sooner you understand that there are hands to pull you over, waiting and outstretched, the quicker you will clear the wall and get on with the rest of the race of life. It is never wise to receive a severe diagnosis from the doctor and hold it to your chest for no one else to see and no one else to help.

As I think through the difficulties of patients and friends who have been struck by illness or accident, I realize that community is not an option, it is a necessity. Some patients have needed transportation to the doctor's office or grocery store. Some needed to have food prepared for them. Others needed someone to listen or laugh with when their diagnosis isolated them from normal life. Some needed a friend to sit with their disabled loved one so they could breathe real air and have their hair done. Many needed training in their new diagnosis so that they could adapt to different physical capacities. Others needed actual help to rebuild their strength and make wounded body parts work better. Many needed guidance to redirect their goals in life and find new hope for the future.

These kinds of help do not automatically appear at our doorstep the morning after the doctor gives us bad news, but they are available. They must be called forth, like my wife, Becky, calls her four Labrador retrievers when they are focused on other business outside.

Some help comes from professionals. I remember recently a woman of fifty who had had her pancreas removed, but then the cancer returned to occupy part of her liver. I was treating her with the appropriate chemotherapy, and the cancer was quite stable, but she continued to lose weight from a cause that I did not initially understand. When I finally realized what was wrong, we asked a nurse to educate her about her poorly controlled diabetes, and she improved dramatically. She needed professional assistance to teach her how to manage the complications of her illness. Proper education from professionals may be very helpful in allowing many to manage their new diagnoses. Some people prefer to slug it out on their own understanding and have to settle for a reduced quality of life. Others do not want to be a bother and remain silent, again not getting the help they need.

There are many forms of professional assistance that patients may access. I have a number of patients who have no way to get to their radiation treatments, but the American Cancer Society provides a free van to transport them. My daughter was able to bounce back from her broken spine not only because of God and the surgeons but also because God and the physical therapists rebuilt her muscles through proper exercise. Some of my patients need counseling for their anxieties or depression; some need an aide in the home to help them with the activities of daily living; some need support groups where others in their condition can share their struggles and ways to overcome them. These types of help and many others are available professionally, and you should ask your doctors how to find them.

Some help comes from professionals; some help comes from family, though sometimes it is most difficult for us to ask for help from those we love at home. Joanna was a patient of mine who needed someone to help her walk every day in order to regain the strength in her legs after a spinal cord injury. "But I can't ask my daughters," she said. "They've got families of their own. I don't want to be a burden to them."

When your children look back, one of the times they will recall with greatest satisfaction will be the time they spent helping you.

I asked her, "Where do you get the most joy in your life, Joanna? Is it when you are getting something or is it when you are helping someone who really needs you?"

"When I'm helping someone who needs me," she answered.

"Then why would you not give your children a chance for that kind of joy? When your children look back on their lives some day, one of the times they will recall with greatest satisfaction will be the time they spent helping you. Even the difficulties will magnify the joy of the memory. Why don't you give them that opportunity?"

Call on your families if they are able. They can provide transportation, food, fellowship, encouragement, and thousands of practical helps we cannot even think of.

When family is not available, friends may supplement support or provide it altogether. Most of the time friends just pop out of the woodwork. When trouble comes they just appear as if a trumpet called them. Thelma works for me moving patients from room to room. Emily is a wonderful eighty-year-old patient with chronic leukemia who has no money or transportation and few family members left. Almost every day Thelma is on the phone with Emily to encourage her. She takes food to Emily's home, and when Emily is sick, Thelma is there to visit. Thelma is a friend who puts her friendship into action.

Sometimes, for various reasons, friends don't step up and offer help when it is needed. This is often because they are either unaware of the need or they don't wish to intrude upon your private difficulties. In these situations, though it is sometimes hard to ask friends for help when you know they have their own burdens, I would recommend you call and ask them to do for you what you would be willing to do for them if they were in your situation. If they are true friends, that probably will take care of most of your needs. It would also be good, if you have a number of friends, to have them over together to let them know of your new problem and to ask them to consider how they might help as a group. I would limit those friends to the ones for whom you would be willing to attend a similar meeting were they to ask you. An alternative would be to call one of your special friends and ask if she or he would be in charge of gathering others to help with your new needs. This seems like a brazen approach for self-sufficient Americans, but this is one instance in which our culture has stolen from us a better standard of community that was present in the early Christian church. "All the believers were one in heart and mind. No one claimed that any of his possessions was his own, but they shared everything they had. . . . There were no needy persons among them. For from time to time those who owned lands or houses sold them, brought the money from the sales and put it at the apostles' feet, and it was distributed to anyone as he had need (Acts 4:32–35).

We need to bring our communities back to this standard, and if we cannot find the courage to ask it from our friends, we should certainly do so from our church. I told you earlier about Katelyn. She was eight years old when she developed leukemia. About one year into her treatment she contracted an infection in her spinal fluid that left her in a coma with little hope from medical science. Our church covered the young girl and her family with prayer and with practical help to the mother and father. The parents had been told that even if she recovered, she would never be normal, never be able to walk and talk again. One month ago, our church watched Katelyn walk slowly across the floor at the front of the church and speak to all of us of her gratitude to God and her church for bringing her through.

Our churches should be there for us. They should be there with prayer. They should also be there to organize and provide whatever practical help is needed with the bad news that the doctor has handed us. If you need meals to get through a crisis time, your fellowship groups should provide them. If you need help watching your invalid loved one so you can make a doctor's appointment or play bridge, your church should provide this. If you are isolated and hopeless, your church members and ministers should be there for you regularly to show you hope and let you know you are loved. When you have overcome the initial shock and crisis of your new diagnosis, the church should be there to provide new avenues of ministry in which you can participate to put the meaning back into your living.

We all must climb over the wall of life; God never meant for any of us to do it alone.

When the doctor brings you bad news, you must not stand in the dirt at the base of the climbing wall alone. You must seek community. You must reach out to those who are unaware of your needs but who are willing to help. We all must climb over the wall of life; God never meant for any of us to do it alone. Who should you call today to help give you a lift?

FIFTEEN

Choose Mission

A few years ago ABC Sports regularly used a line something like this: "From the thrill of victory to the agony of defeat." That's true not only in athletic competitions; it's true in life. We win and we lose. For most of us, the thrill of victory in life comes from personal achievement, recreational pleasure, touching beauty, good health, good friends, a happy family. The agony of defeat hits us in personal failure, surroundings of ugliness, absence of pleasure, loneliness, an unhappy family, loss of health. The ultimate agony of defeat, to us, is death. How do we face what we would call the agony of defeat and find peace within it? Many of our great biblical heroes did. Remember Elijah?

Elijah felt like a young boy in spite of his arthritis. He actually attempted to jump up in the air and click his heels as he thanked God for the new youth in his heart. He grinned as he remembered the day before when he had challenged the people of Israel on Mount Carmel, "How long will you waver between two opinions? If the Lord is God, follow him; but if Baal is God, follow him" (1 Kings 18:21). He then had challenged the prophets of Baal to a duel, their god against his. And God had come through! Fire from heaven, all the prophets of Baal destroyed, and "When all the people saw this, they fell prostrate and cried, 'The Lord—he is God! The Lord—he is God!'" (1 Kings 18:39). What a marvelous victory.

Then Elijah received the message from Jezebel, and joy drained from his body and his limbs trembled. Jezebel's message said he would die before tomorrow. From joy and life to fear and death within one moment.

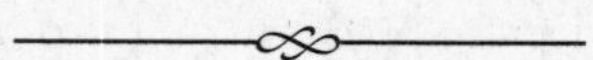

How many of us have received that message of a debilitating illness by mail, by phone, or sitting across from the strained face of a doctor? How does one cope? What can one do? "Elijah was afraid and ran for his life" (1 Kings 19:3). But Elijah recovered from his fear and returned to a life that mattered. He not only came out of his self-absorption; he found that he still had a mission waiting for him. What were the steps in his transformation between total absorption with his own troubles to a life that would count again?

After running for days, Elijah found himself in the desert. Though he was running from death, he had also given up. "He came to a broom tree, sat down under it and prayed that he might die. 'I have had enough, Lord,' he said. 'Take my life; I am no better than my ancestors'" (1 Kings 19:4). Then the Lord began to work, one step at a time:

Step 1: Rest in the Lord

> Then he lay down under the tree and fell asleep. All at once an angel touched him and said, "Get up and eat." He looked around, and there by his head was a cake of bread baked over hot coals, and a jar of water. He ate and drank and then lay down again.
>
> The angel of the Lord came back a second time and touched him and said, "Get up and eat, for the journey is too much for you." So he got up and ate and drank.
>
> —1 Kings 19:5–8

The journey was too much for Elijah. The journey is too much for us as we face our suffering in the future. Sometimes we just have to drop everything and rest. The Sunday after the tragedy of sixteen murdered children in his parish, the minister of Dunblane Cathedral in Scotland said (and I paraphrase), "We've had enough attention. We've had enough questions. Now what we need is time and space and silence to grieve."

Have you ever had a child who wanted something so badly, and when it didn't happen, he came to you broken and crying? When children are really broken, it's not the time for discussion, analysis, and planning; it is time for them to crawl into your lap and be held in your arms. They need "time and space and silence."

I remember with tears Sherry, a woman of fifty whom we thought had been cured of breast cancer. I remember the day I felt her liver and discovered it to be hard and enlarged. I felt certain it was cancer but did not tell her at first. I remember the next day when she returned for her CT report, and I told her it was cancer. From that second on, she knew she was going to die. She fell into my arms and simply cried—no words.

There comes a time after the initial discovery of a life-changing illness that it is necessary to grieve and to fall in someone's arms and simply rest.

When we rest, it is critical that we choose arms that can hold us well. We need to rest in the arms of those who love us, and we need them to understand that at times we just need holding. But the arms of those we love can hold us only so long, so we also must crawl into the arms of the one who is strong enough to carry us through all circumstances. And that one promises: "I will never leave you nor forsake you" (Josh. 1:5).

Step 2: Return to Your Spiritual Roots

> Strengthened by that food, he traveled forty days and forty nights until he reached Horeb, the mountain of God.
>
> —1 Kings 19:8

Sometimes it is we who have left God. We suddenly need him desperately, and we don't know where to find him. Elijah felt the same way and searched for God. He went back to Horeb, the place where

Israel had found God in the wilderness, the place of the burning bush, the place where God had given them the Law. In the midst of our pain, if we know we need God but cannot find him, we must go back to where we knew him before—a time in our memory or an actual location where we knew God was at that time. Then in those memories, realize that God has not changed. In those memories, rest and pray and read his Word, and we will find that the God we cannot seem to find picks us up and carries us.

In prison before he was killed by the Nazis, Dietrich Bonhoeffer wrote a poem entitled "Who Am I?" It describes the thoughts that ran through his mind in prison while he was awaiting death. He speaks of all the confusion twisting through his mind. He settles his tormented questions with the lines, "Who am I? They mock me, these lonely questions of mine. Whoever I am, thou knowest, O God, I am thine."[1]

There comes a time as we face our personal tragedies that it all is too much for us. At that time we, like Elijah and Bonhoeffer, must seek God, then very simply crawl into his arms and rest.

STEP 3: REVEAL YOUR HEART TO THE LORD

> And the word of the LORD came to him: "What are you doing here, Elijah?"
>
> He replied, "I have been very zealous for the LORD God Almighty. The Israelites have rejected your covenant, broken down your altars, and put your prophets to death with the sword. I am the only one left, and now they are trying to kill me too."
>
> —1 KINGS 19:9–10

When children get to their teenage years, it seems they don't want to communicate. We parents know they are hurting, but we can't force them to talk so that we can help. When facing the prospect of a serious illness, we can be like those teenagers. We shut up in our discouragement and fail to tell it all to the only one who can fix it. When we are broken, God wants to hear from us. He wants our praise and trust when that's what we feel, but he also wants our brokenness and discouragement when that is what we feel. God doesn't need to hear your problems in order to know what to do, but you need to speak them to him or else your ears will be plugged with your own stifled cries, and you will never get to step 4.

STEP 4: LISTEN FOR THE WHISPER

> The LORD said, "Go out and stand on the mountain in the presence of the LORD, for the LORD is about to pass by."
>
> Then a great and powerful wind tore the mountains apart and shattered the rocks before the LORD, but the LORD was not in the wind. After the wind there was an earthquake, but the LORD was not in the earthquake. After the earthquake came a fire, but the LORD was not in the fire. And after the fire came a gentle whisper. When Elijah heard it, he pulled his cloak over his face and went out and stood at the mouth of the cave.
>
> —1 KINGS 19:11–13

Have you ever heard the whisper of God? I can recall two occasions related to my mission work in Nigeria when God whispered, and it made all the difference in the world. The first was in the days prior to leaving for Nigeria when there was a great struggle within me. I knew God had called me to that place, but I couldn't bear the thought of leaving home and uprooting my wife and children for a life with no security. One day I was at a family outing at a campground when I finally said to myself, "No, I can't do it!" Immediately there came a voice without volume but with words that were clear, "Yes, you will do it." And I knew it was the whisper of God, and I lost all my anxiety, and I went to the mission field.

The second time I heard his whisper was on the opposite end of my time in Africa. We had planned Africa as a career and Eku as our home, but my wife's health failed, and I knew we had to go home for her sake. I was tormented because I didn't want to leave the place where God's mission was so clear to me. It was dark, and I was sitting on a cheap lawn chair under our belebo tree. I was crying in my loss. Then above me between the trees appeared (at least to my mind) a vague figure and a voice without sound that said clearly, "It's all right, Al. Take her home." And I did. It was the whisper of God, and it was the will of God, and it was all right.

Events and time have convinced me that these were not delusions or early schizophrenia but truly God speaking to me. He loves his people. He wants to speak into our lives. But we must listen.

These are rather stark examples in my own life of the whisper of God. Most of the time in my life, however, God's whisper has not come with audible words but with words on the pages of the Bible, or words from the mouth of a loved one, or events that show me he is near. The problem is that we can sometimes hear that whisper and not recognize it as his—unless we are listening for him to speak.

As we read in Genesis 22, Abraham climbed the hill with his only son, Isaac, expecting to sacrifice his son on the altar of God. God had spoken clearly, and Abraham obeyed. But all the way he was listening, probably thinking, "Surely God will speak again." Step by step, he listened; as he tied his beloved child to the altar, he listened; as he raised his knife to slay the one he loved most in all the world, he listened; and because he listened, he heard God speak, and Isaac was spared.

Even as you take the steps through the door of your new diagnosis, you must listen for God. You may not have the answers to the questions that torment you about your family, your suffering, and your fear of the temporary darkness ahead. But if you listen, he will speak—in some way, through someone, on some page, or in some event. And if you listen for him, you will know it is God, and you can go on.

STEP 5: RETURN TO WORK

> The LORD said to him, "Go back the way you came, and go to the Desert of Damascus. When you get there, anoint Hazael king over Aram. Also, anoint Jehu son of Nimshi king over Israel, and anoint Elisha son of Shaphat from Abel Meholah to succeed you as prophet. Jehu will put to death any who escape the sword of Hazael, and Elisha will put to death any who escape the sword of Jehu."
>
> —1 KINGS 19:15–17

Elijah may have been expecting God to stroke him and pity him, but God had already comforted and fed Elijah. Here God says, "You get back to work. I'll take care of things." There comes a time in our lives after the shock of our bad news that we have to get back to the business of living. We were placed here on earth with a purpose in God's mind and given a certain number of days to complete it. "For we are God's workmanship, created in Christ Jesus to do good works, which God prepared in advance for us to do" (Eph. 2:10).

We can quit this life, quit our work, and leave our job unfinished as soon as we face difficulties, or we can pick ourselves up, dust ourselves off, put our hands to the plow, and work until our job is done. After the tears, we must once again focus on what God has brought us here to do.

We treated Myra Max very aggressively when she was discovered to have lymphoma, but it became clear she would not be cured. We therefore stopped treatment and left her in the Lord's hands. He took her lymphoma away. Myra printed for my office a thousand copies of a poem distributed at the memorial service of a Christian named Dan Richardson, who died of cancer. I'd like to share it with you:

> Cancer is so limited . . .
> It cannot cripple love,
> It cannot shatter hope,
> It cannot corrode faith,
> It cannot eat away peace,
> It cannot destroy confidence,
> It cannot kill friendship,
> It cannot shut out memories,
> It cannot silence courage,
> It cannot invade the soul,
> It cannot reduce eternal life,
> It cannot quench the Spirit,
> It cannot lessen the power of the resurrection.
>
> —AUTHOR UNKNOWN

More people who come to me with cancer have been blessed by the poem that Myra printed than by any words of comfort I have spoken.

Marti had slowly progressing colon cancer in her liver. Over her last year of life, when she became too weak to get out, she began painting little stand-up cards with beautiful flowers and verses of hope from God's Word and gave them away to those who needed comfort. Murray Alexander, with metastatic renal cancer, is not sure when or whether the cancer in his liver will return, but he's not sitting still. He has just returned from a mission trip to Spain. These patients, with their illnesses, rose up from their despair, looked out the window, and said, "There's still daylight left; I'll get a bit more done before the sunset." You can look at the remainder of your life either as wasted time to use in dying or as God-given time to complete your mission. God told Elijah, "Get back to work. I'll take care of things."

You can look at the remainder of your life either as wasted time to use in dying or as God-given time to complete your mission.

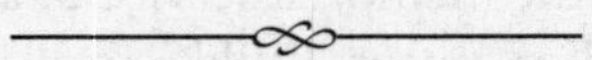

One day when driving home from work I heard a commentator on public radio discuss the discovery of a Neanderthal man in the ice of a glacier. The commentator stated, "You know, there is something very peaceful about a body frozen for five thousand years." Death can be much like a snake rising in our path, where just the sight of it, without its bite, may leave us involuntarily frozen, like the Neanderthal, and unable to continue with life. God tells us in our fear to get up and keep living. Serious illness is something we should pass through while walking the road of life, not an ocean that catches us in its rising tide while we lay immobile on its banks. Larry Sanders understood this.

A young Christian nurse in my clinic stopped me at the nurse's station one day and told me what she called "a neat missionary story" about her father, Larry Sanders:

> My father died a few years ago. He was a patient here with a sarcoma. Before he developed cancer, he

loved to go on mission trips and returned over and over again to Guyana. Near the end of his life with cancer, at forty-nine years of age, he had had one leg amputated and was sick all the time from the treatment, but he badly wanted to make another mission trip to Guyana. We all were afraid for him and tried to talk him out of it, but he went anyway. It was difficult for him, but he made it all right and returned, then died of his cancer.

This past Christmas, a friend of mine called me. She had moved from Memphis to Benton, Arkansas. She started a Bible study with the women there. One day they were all giving their personal testimonies, when a young woman with an accent told her story to the group.

"I came to know the Lord when I lived in Guyana a few years ago. There was a missionary who kept coming there, telling us about Jesus. My parents accepted Jesus as their Savior and were always talking about Jesus and reading the Bible. But I just couldn't believe. I couldn't accept what they were saying until one day that missionary returned. I saw him walking up the mountain, sick, and with only one leg, and I knew that if Jesus was important enough for that missionary to come to us as sick as he was, then I needed to make him my Savior too."

This young woman from Guyana will live with God forever because Larry Sanders did not quit. God told Paul in the midst of his discouragement, "Get up and keep speaking." As Larry Sanders faced death with cancer, he heard the same message from God, got up on one leg, and accomplished things of eternal significance. As you consider your future, however difficult it will be, will you choose to do the same?

SIXTEEN

Choose to Hold On

Sometimes in spite of all our prayer and all our trust, the doctor's bad news is still more than we can face. At those times it is okay just to hold on.

In a September 1996 comic strip, John Hart used his cartoon character B. C. to give us all a good word of advice. His words of wisdom were: "Never get on a roller coaster that leaves full and comes back half empty."

Good advice. Many of us have lived lives like a roller coaster: the slow, boring, uphill climbs; the fear of uncertainty as we reach the top of the rails and see nothing but the sky; the wildness of the downhill ride. Remember what you did the last time you rode a roller coaster? My ten-year-old son would laugh with his hands raised high, but if you are like me, you *held on*. Like me, you held on because you were afraid of falling out.

Facing serious illness is like riding a roller coaster: endless days of drudgery without the energy or desire to accomplish anything, that great fear of uncertainty as you reach the top of the rails and see nothing but the endless night sky, that wild and sometimes painful ride downhill as we are smashed against the side of our car with every sharp turn.

The writer of Hebrews had never seen a roller coaster but had ridden life and faced death as much as any of us. He knew the necessity of holding on:

> But Christ is faithful as a son over God's house. And we are his house, if we ***hold on*** to our courage and the hope of which we boast.
>
> —HEBREWS 3:6 (ITALICS MINE)

> We have come to share in Christ if ***we hold firmly*** till the end the confidence we had at first.
>
> —HEBREWS 3:14 (ITALICS MINE)

As you consider the doctor's bad news, hold on. Holding on is action and requires energy. It is something you *do.* Though not sufficient in itself to keep you safe, God has told you to do so. It is your responsibility in partnership with him as together you work out the mission of life to which he has called you. Assuming this is true, what is it that Christians can hold on to as they look at tough times in their future?

HOLD ON TO MEMORIES OF HIS PRESENCE AND ACTION IN OUR LIVES

I'll never forget the moment Catherine Ekhator handed me two-and-a-half-dozen eggs in Benin City, Nigeria. It was August 1984. A patient named Matthew was dying on the medicine ward at Eku Hospital. He badly needed blood, but there was little to be found. A missionary nurse, Jackie Legg, had his blood type and gave one unit; but Matthew needed at least two units to survive. There was a young Nigerian nursing student who was willing to give, but only if we gave him a dozen eggs to restore his power after the bloodletting. I told my wife, Becky, of the problem, and she offered our last dozen eggs. We needed those eggs badly as there were none to be found in the stores, and we had two children. Nevertheless, Becky was willing to give up the eggs for my patient. Matthew received the blood, later recovered, and accepted Jesus Christ as his Savior. My kids were left without eggs.

The Sunday after the transfusion, I was asked to speak at a church in Benin City. After the service I visited the pastor's house for lunch. As I left that family and walked to my car, the pastor's wife, Catherine, told me to wait. She entered her house and returned with a gift for my wife—two-and-a-half-dozen eggs. Though Catherine knew nothing of our need or our sacrifice, God knew of both. He was there that day, and I will hold on to that memory of God's presence and action whenever I face the needs and sacrifices of the future. Reach back and grab the days when you saw God in action in your life, then hold on.

HOLD ON TO HIS WORD

How much Scripture have I kept in my mind that I can return to in time of need? There was a time in my youth when I memorized large sections of God's Word. As much work as it was then, those are now the Scriptures to which I return when I face the storms of life. As the writer of Hebrews knew, God's Word is alive and cuts right to the center of our existence (Heb. 4:12–13).

I walked into Mr. Brocietti's room early one morning to find him reading the Bible. Mr. Brocietti had terminal pancreatic cancer and was admitted to the hospital for a nerve block to help control his pain. He showed me the verses he was reading in the twenty-first chapter of Revelation, which describe the future Jerusalem. "It's a beautiful place isn't it?" he asked, smiling at me, the doctor who had told him he was going to die. God's Word can bring hope to our lives when no one else can.

HOLD ON TO THE KNOWLEDGE THAT I AM A SINNER, SAVED

My brother-in-law went through a difficult time of depression soon after marrying my sister and moving to Oregon. During that time he said the words of a popular song kept ringing in his ears: "You're no good, you're no good, you're no good; Baby, you're no good." He felt the artist was singing to him.

It is not healthy for any of us to continually beat ourselves into depression with our failings, but we must not as Christians ever forget whence we came. It is the understanding of our sinfulness that helps us most to remove the coat of anger and resentment that comes when we perceive undeserved difficulties. Death for us is justice, and it is only the grace of God that gives us eternal life beyond.

Hold on to the Knowledge That He Is Present

The people of Israel had lost their great leader, Moses. Now they looked across the Jordan River at a new and strange land, full of unknown danger and enemies who could destroy them. Moses had laid his hands on Joshua to lead the Israelites into this new and dangerous land. Joshua may have been afraid, but he knew he was not alone. God came to him in private three days before the river crossing. "As I was with Moses, so I will be with you; I will never leave you nor forsake you" (Josh. 1:5). Neither life nor death can keep us from his presence.

David knew it:

> Where can I go from your Spirit?
> Where can I flee from your presence?
> If I go to the heavens, you are there;
> if I make my bed in the depths, you are there.
> If I rise on the wings of the dawn,
> if I settle on the far side of the sea,
> even there your hand will guide me,
> your right hand will hold me fast.
> If I say, "Surely the darkness will hide me
> and the light become night around me,"
> even the darkness will not be dark to you;
> the night will shine like the day,
> for darkness is as light to you.
>
> —Psalm 139:7–12

Paul knew it: "For I am convinced that neither death nor life, neither angels nor demons, neither the present nor the future, nor any powers, neither height nor depth, nor anything else in all creation, will be able to separate us from the love of God that is Christ Jesus our Lord" (Rom. 8:38–39).

Mr. Leflin knew it: Early in his illness, after he had discovered he was going to die from cancer, he was very discouraged and depressed. He was up alone one night in that state of depression when he felt a touch on his shoulder. He looked around and saw no one, but he knew that God was there. He felt the peace of God enter his life at that moment and wash away his despair. He lost his fear. He lost his depression. His family says he became a different man. He got out of his bed and became part of the family instead of just lying there waiting to die. He said he was ready for the end of his life but would be happy to live as long as God's peace remained with him.

Jesus said it: "And surely I am with you always, to the very end of the age" (Matt. 28:20).

You do not face your future alone. The one who died for you and has the power to save you for eternity will never leave your side. Never.

Hold on to the Knowledge That He Will Get You Through

Becky and Janice were driving back from grocery shopping in Warre. They had not anticipated the *juju* festival as they left the highway and drove the rutted, muddy road through the backside of Eku to get to our compound. Their three children played in the back seat of the Nigerian-made station wagon, oblivious to the men around the next bend in the road. As they made that turn, a mob of half-naked local men with painted faces and headdresses attacked the car, some beating on it, others waving machetes. They demanded money to let Becky, Janice, and the children pass. There was real fear in her heart as Becky told the drunken men that she worked at Eku Hospital. When she mentioned the hospital, a leader stepped forward and told the mob to let Becky pass. She drove home safely without further threat.

Becky made it through the drunken mob because she was connected to the hospital. We, too, are connected. We are connected to the one who holds the universe in his hands, and he promises to get us through the fearful faces of sickness, injury, and death that rise up before us. He promises to get us home.

> And this is the will of him who sent me, that I shall lose none of all that he has given me, but raise them up at the last day. For my Father's will is that everyone who looks to the Son and believes in him shall have eternal life, and I will raise him up at the last day.
>
> —John 6:39–40

> I have told you these things, so that in me you may have peace. In this world you will have trouble. But take heart! I have overcome the world.
>
> —John 16:33

Just as Becky passed through the drunken mob at Eku and made it home safely, you will pass through the threatening presence of your illness and make it home as well, because Christ has promised that with his work and his power, nothing can stand in your way.

Hold on to Each Other

As we have said earlier, God never intended us to be solo Christians fighting through life and death in Satan's world on our own. He has given us the church, and Paul says the church is there for us to hold on to when the waves are driving us under:

> Make every effort to keep the unity of the Spirit through the bond of peace. There is one body and one Spirit—just as you were called to one hope when you were called—one Lord, one faith, one baptism; one God and Father of all, who is over all and through all and in all. Then we will no longer . . . be infants, tossed back and forth by the waves, and blown here and there by every wind of teaching and by the cunning and craftiness of men in their deceitful scheming. Instead, speaking the truth in love, we will in all things grow up into him who is the Head, that is, Christ. From him the whole body, joined and held together by every supporting ligament, grows and builds itself up in love, as each part does its work.
>
> —Ephesians 4:3–6, 14–16

We live this life and face death as individuals in a boat on a stormy sea. Each of us, in our time, is tossed overboard, and we find ourselves floundering in the waves and wind. When I am in the brine, I need you to throw me the lifeline, and when you are there, I need to toss the line to you. This is the way God planned the church to be. We dare not face serious illness or death as individuals who refuse to grab the lifeline that is thrown to us unless we wish to suffer far more than God intended.

So the writer of Hebrews encourages us to hold on. When we face our brokenness, we must hold on. But we are human, weak, and tired, and sometimes we just let go. What then? What happens if you fail to hold on to the securities that God has provided for you for this time? If you let go, will you fall from the boat with the next wave?

What happens in a roller coaster ride if you let go? Do you fall out? No. You will slide and hit the sides of the car on the turns and hurt, cry, and possibly throw up, but you will not fall out. You will not fall out because, at the beginning of the ride, the conductor locked a bar across your lap, and that bar will hold you in the car. Just so, your ride through life as a Christian began when you gave your ticket to the Conductor of life. You accepted Christ as your Savior and climbed in the car. When you did, before the ride started, the Conductor laid his Cross as a safety belt across your lap that will never let you fall out. If you let go, you may get beat up pretty badly, you may forget why you got on, and you may lose the joy of the ride, but you will never fall out.

The Conductor has laid his Cross over your lap, and you will never fall out.

Hold on and feel the joy of the ride, even when it might be painful. Realize that holding on is what maximizes joy and minimizes pain. Realize, however, that ultimately it is not your holding on but his Cross that will bring you safely to the conclusion of the ride.

SEVENTEEN

Choose to Overcome

Peter could not believe what he had just heard. Jesus had just informed the disciples that he was leaving them, and he had picked the Passover feast to do so. Peter knew it was getting tough for his Master, but he never thought of him as one who would give up and leave. Peter looked into his eyes, sadder than he had seen them before, and asked, "'Lord, where are you going?' Jesus replied, 'Where I am going, you cannot follow now, but you will follow later.' Peter asked, 'Lord, why can't I follow you now? I will lay down my life for you.' Then Jesus answered, 'Will you really lay down your life for me? I tell you the truth, before the rooster crows, you will disown me three times!'" (John 13:36–38).

Peter proved himself in the garden where Jesus prayed. They came to take Jesus away, and with no thought for his own life, Peter drew his sword and attacked. To his surprise, Jesus rebuked him, "Put your sword away! Shall I not drink the cup the Father has given me?" (John 18:11).

Then they led Jesus away as a prisoner. Peter followed from a distance. He had done what he said he would do. He had laid his life on the line for Jesus, and Jesus had rejected his action. What more could he do?

> "You are not one of his disciples, are you?" the girl at the door asked Peter.
>
> He replied, "I am not."
>
> It was cold. . . .
>
> As Simon Peter stood warming himself, he was asked, "You are not one of his disciples, are you?"
>
> He denied it, saying, "I am not."
>
> One of the high priest's servants, a relative of the man whose ear Peter had cut off, challenged him, "Didn't I see you with him in the olive grove?" Again Peter denied it, and at that moment a rooster began to crow.
>
> —John 18:17–18, 25–27

There are many ways for Christians to deny Christ. Even those who love him most and feel they would die for him, like Peter, encounter circumstances in life that sometimes beat them down to the point that their resolve is gone. When asked publicly, Peter denied he knew Jesus. Few of us would do that today in our free Western society. But there are other ways to deny him. When confronted with serious health problems, many who have been comfortable in their faith during good times deny God in despair. They deny God not by speaking against him but by refusing to let him be who he really is: Savior, Comforter, King of kings, Creator, Alpha and Omega, the Beginning and End of all things. They deny God by letting go of him and frantically grasping at all the props the world offers as their only hope. Eventually they realize it is all to no avail, and they face death utterly alone, having let go of the one person who could carry them through safely.

Reasons Why We May Deny God

Why does that happen? Why do people who talk about God and attend church sometimes shut off his presence when confronted with life-threatening illness? It has been my experience that some of the most frantic seekers of quack remedies for fatal illnesses are Bible-believing Christians who have the least to lose with death. Are they denying God his lordship? Are these Christians, who refuse to be comforted and who lie in fear and anger as death approaches, denying God the place he demands in our hearts? There are a number of reasons why men and women dedicated to God may deny him in this way when they hear the doctor's bad news.

1. Fear paralyzes us. When I was young, my father served a stint as camp doctor at a Boy Scout camp in Arkansas—a cheap family vacation. I remember the experience at Camp KiaKima when walking the wooded trail by the river. A snake appeared suddenly in the middle of the path, coiled with its head up, ready to strike. I froze and was absolutely unable to move until long after the snake had slid away.

The fear of broken health may have paralyzed you. Even when you normally would desperately reach for God, you cannot do so in your frozenness, and you may have dropped his hand from yours.

2. Pride barricades us. We often go through life paying lip service and playing ritual games with God, all the while being satisfied with our own security system. When faced with a health problem we cannot control, we continue in our usual mode, building higher walls to keep death away, and in doing so, confident in our own ability, we leave God on the outside of the wall.

3. Confusion distorts us. Peter laid his life on the line and did what he knew was best when he struck with the sword to defend Jesus. Then Jesus rebuked him! Peter didn't know why. Confusion followed and left Peter no clear footing to keep from sliding when pressed by accusations. We think sometimes we understand God and, having figured him out, know how to get what we need in life. Then the bottom falls out, and our previous understanding of how to push God's buttons doesn't hold up. We think, what good is God to me? Confusion.

4. Distraction blinds us. In the courtyard, Peter was focused on solving Jesus' problem of being arrested. With that focus, it made no sense to admit knowing him. That would not help his Master. Once before

Peter had focused on the wrong thing. Jesus had told Peter to walk to him upon the water. As long as Peter focused on Jesus, his feet skimmed the surface, but when he peered into the waves and lost sight of Jesus, he began to sink and drown. When the thought of a serious illness becomes real in our lives, we, too, often will divert our gaze from God and peer into those dark waves. Sometimes we fail to look up again until we are drowning.

5. *Inertia carries us.* Peter's first denial was due to his confusion, but the second and third were propelled by the first. Once he started lying, the lies became easier and more necessary. You may be caught up in a life that depends on the world, not on your God. When broken health comes into the picture, the world's conveyor belt just keeps you moving, and in the crisis you cannot figure out how to get off the world's conveyor belt and get over to God.

6. *Aloneness weakens us.* With Jesus beside him, Peter was a lion. When alone, Peter's courage vanished. Facing an illness that changes who we are in the eyes of the world is one of the loneliest things we do. If you have lived your life before with only a superficial relationship to God, it may seem uncomfortable to let him in on this last intense personal experience, so you may not make the effort.

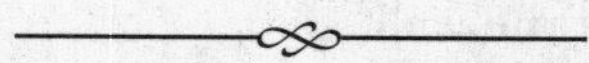

These six phenomena may deny God the access to your life that he desires in order for him to carry you through your sickness with peace. But even with these obstacles, God has given you the tools necessary to overcome them and to allow him to be who he wants to be in this greatest of all your trials. How do you climb over these obstacles to reach God's presence?

Overcoming Fear

If we are to avoid the shock of serious illness, we must first accept such illness as part of life's package from the beginning. "There is a time for everything, and a season for every activity under heaven: a time to be born and a time to die" (Eccl. 3:1–2). Most people don't ever admit that sickness and death are a part of life until they get stuck on the tracks with the train coming. We need to understand this fact of life early; then the fear that comes from surprise vanishes.

Second, we must know whose hands are holding us. We are afraid because we fear we will fall into nothingness or into an accidental world. We are not convinced that God's hands can hold us when ours have become so weak. We must have confidence that the hands that hold us are indeed the hands of God, which will not let us go. "And this is the will of him who sent me, that I shall lose none of all that he has given me, but raise them up at the last day" (John 6:39). "I know whom I have believed, and am persuaded that he is able to guard that which I have committed unto him against that day" (2 Tim. 1:12 ASV). We can be confident that we are in the hands of God and that his hands never lose their grip.

My favorite psychiatrist, David Allen, told this story at a deacons' banquet at my church a few years ago:

One warm summer day a young boy was walking along the bank of the Mississippi River when he came upon a tramp sitting under a shade tree watching the boats go by. Typical for his age, the boy sat down beside the man and began asking questions. Glad to have some company, the tramp chatted with the boy about unimportant things. As they were talking, a riverboat came into view and seemed like it would pass them on the river.

The boy rose and began waving his hands frantically, jumping up and down, calling to the boat. The tramp thought this to be silly behavior and laughed at the boy. "You're crazy, boy," he said. "There's no way that boat is going to pay any attention to you."

But the boy kept jumping and waving until finally, to the tramp's surprise, the riverboat began to turn. It headed for the bank, pulled right up into the mud, and let down its plank. The tramp sat dumbfounded as the boy walked up the plank and jumped into the boat. Then, as the boat was backing away from the shore, the boy cupped his hands and shouted over the engines, "I knew it would come. The captain is my daddy."

The fullness of life may seem to be drifting past, with you sitting wounded on the side. You may be afraid that goodness and value are moving beyond your reach, that the night will come and find you on the riverbank alone. Not so. The Captain of life is your Daddy. God sees you where you are, and he will not leave you stranded.

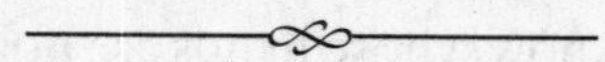

Finally, in order to overcome our fear of suffering, we must realize that when we do suffer, our anguish is not wasted. Paul was isolated under house arrest in Rome before he died, and yet he wrote, "Now I want you to know, brothers, that what has happened to me has really served to advance the gospel" (Phil. 1:12). Fear is easier to bear if we know that good comes out of our suffering. God does not usually cause our suffering in order to bring good, but he always uses our suffering to create good. We can be brave and know that when we walk with him through serious illness, he will use that walk for great things.

Overcoming Pride

Stop, look around, and realize that even if your systems beat the odds and even if you stretch out your life a bit longer by using your skills, you are waging a war for merely months or years within the time frame of eternity. If you win the brief battle by your skills, that means almost nothing in the true war. Only God fights in the time frame of eternity. Let us not become isolated in our own little battle away from our General. Even those who fought hardest at Little Big Horn did die in the end. "This is the evil in everything that happens under the sun: The same destiny overtakes all" (Eccl. 9:3).

Overcoming Confusion

Accept the truth that you don't have to understand. David says of God's understanding, "Such knowledge is too wonderful for me, too lofty for me to attain" (Ps. 139:6). In the book of Isaiah, God speaks: "'For my thoughts are not your thoughts, neither are your ways my ways,' declares the Lord. 'As the heavens are higher than the earth, so are my ways higher than your ways and my thoughts than your thoughts" (Isa. 55:8–9). Accept the fact that the rationale of suffering, death, and eternity are beyond your grasp. Don't force yourself to live with the lights off because you cannot understand electricity.

Often our confusion centers on the questions, "Why doesn't God come through for me when I ask? Does he really love me?" These questions rise to the surface whether we wish them to or not—and I believe they can be answered. If God is all-knowing and all-powerful, and if he really loves us, then I am convinced that we do not suffer in this world unless *God has planned for us, in our suffering, a purpose that is greater than our pain*. Sometimes we discover that purpose even before we get to heaven.

Jennifer Hanks is a patient of mine with two small children. She is doing well now but had a very difficult six months of treatment lasting through the summer. Because of her illness her children lost most of their summer fun. Just prior to school starting, things were getting better and Jennifer prepared a holiday weekend at Pickwick Lake. Her eight-year-old son was ecstatic that some fun was finally coming again into his life. He prayed daily that God would not let this trip be canceled like so many other events of the last six months. The weekend came, the rain poured down, and the trip was canceled.

Believing that God should have listened to his prayers, the boy told his mother, "I asked God to let us go. Why didn't he answer?"

With wisdom well beyond mine, Jennifer replied, "God did answer. His answer was 'no.' But he said 'no' to Pickwick so he could say 'yes' someday to something better."

When Jennifer was consoling her son, she did not know that some of her friends had put her name and her kids' names in to the Make a Wish Foundation. Soon after the failed trip to the lake, she and her two boys were awarded a fully paid trip to Disneyland.

"Don't you see?" she told her son, "God said 'no' to Pickwick so he could say 'yes' to Disneyland."

That's the way it is with God. Though you may be confused by his answer to your present plea, you can be confident that within his "no" there is always a purpose greater than your pain, and that someday he will be saying "yes" to something better.

We are more likely to be confused by God if we never listen for him to speak. That listening comes with prayer and with the study of his Word. Sometimes the answers for our questions about life and death are available, and we don't know them because we do not seek them. Sometimes this ignorance leads to fear, whereas knowledge would have set us free from that fear. "If you hold to my teaching, you are really my disciples. Then you will know the truth, and the truth will set you free" (John 8:31–32). Much of the knowledge that will free us from the fear of suffering is readily available in his Word, yet we choose to remain confused and afraid rather than study.

Overcoming Distraction

How can we walk through this world focused on the face of God when desperate issues demand our full attention? It takes incredible discipline to study his Word, pray regularly, and seek his face each day when you are worried about the bad news your doctor has given you and every waking moment is spent in trying to find a way out, a treatment, a cure. But we have an incredible God who says, "If you look for me in earnest, you will find me when you seek me" (Jer. 29:13 NLT). Take him at his Word, turn your heart to him, spend time with him, and soon you will see him lifting you up like Peter walking on top of the angry waves.

Overcoming Aloneness

In order to combat the fear that comes from the desperation of being alone, you must:

1. *Choose to be his:* "Behold, I stand at the door and knock; if anyone hears . . . My voice and opens the door, I will come in . . . and will eat with him, and he with Me" (Rev. 3:20 AMPLIFIED).
2. *Realize he is with you:* "And lo, I am with you always, even unto the end of the world" (Matt. 28:20 ASV).
3. *Stay in communication with him:* "Do not be anxious about anything, but in everything, by prayer and petition, with thanksgiving, present your requests to God.

And the peace of God, which transcends all understanding, will guard your hearts and your minds in Christ Jesus" (Phil. 4:6–7).

4. *Seek community:* Peter began to heal the wounds of his denial when he returned to his friends and together they awaited the unknown. God has not made us to stand alone in our pain.

Jim is seventy-six years old and has chronic leukemia. One day I told him that he may need therapy soon in order to continue living.

"I don't want that," he said.

"Why not?" I asked.

"I live alone. All my buddies are gone. I've got no family. All I do every day is watch television alone."

"Jim," I said, "you need community in order to make your life worth living again, and then we can talk about making you live longer. You need people to talk to and friends to do things with. Is there anyone? Are you a member of a church?"

"No, I never was religious. Besides, I don't have anything in common with anyone now that all my Army buddies are gone. I'd have nothing to talk about."

"But that's the point, Jim. Your life has been different from those around you. You've got plenty to talk about. If you share your experiences with others, they will benefit from your being there. You can make a contribution by sharing your life with people who have never imagined what you and your Army buddies went through together."

"I see what you mean," Jim said. "Perhaps."

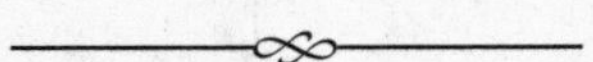

As we face broken health, Satan would steal the peace that should be ours by having us deny God the place in our lives where God wishes to work. We are attacked with fear, pride, distraction, inertia, and aloneness. But God understands these forces and can overcome them. We need merely to follow his guidelines to open the door. As God enters, fear will exit through the same door.

EIGHTEEN

Anticipate Your Future

One Saturday morning this past summer I got it in my head to run six miles. This was a peculiar thought, but it would not let go. I was in the habit of running three miles when I felt like it once or twice a week, and this would be twice my distance. Besides that, it was ninety degrees outside. It was a peculiar and foolish thing to do, but, always having been one who followed impulse rather than reason, I started out. The first three miles were great. The fourth was a challenge, with my clothes soaked in sweat, the sun beating down on my shoulders, and the thought that I was doing something extraordinary urging me on. The fifth mile was unpleasant, with my tongue like cotton and the Memphis humidity thick as a blanket. The fun and excitement of the run had vanished. The last mile was nearly impossible. My hips ached, and I could barely hold my head up in the heat. I ran from tree to tree, even dodging out of my way for a few seconds of shade.

There was no way I was going to make it through that final mile until I thought of the swimming pool. We have a small pool in the backyard with cool water in the summer's heat. When I began to think of diving into that refreshing pool at the end of my run, my legs found new strength. I closed my eyes as step by step I drew closer and felt the rush of that water over my parched skin. For that last mile of my run, it was the vision of the pool that kept me going. Even better than the vision was the reality as I finally fell into the wonderful coolness I had dreamed of while running.

I am not knowledgeable regarding the understanding of the afterlife in other religious faiths, but those of us who are Christians can't lose. We start off running the race of life with energy and excitement. Somewhere along the way we feel pain and fatigue as life grows heavy. Toward the end of our race, we see death with all of its fears and difficulties. In spite of that discovery we need to continue; we need to run each lap with God at our side. Sometimes, however, the pain, the fatigue, and the despair are so great that we would faint in spite of all the help God gives us. That's the time to think of the pool at the end of the run. That's the time to realize there is a heaven. The critical illness or injury we face may or may not bring us close enough to death to see it in our near future. But all of us know that death is ahead, and that knowledge colors how we handle the medical difficulties we now face. We need to settle the question of death by setting our eyes beyond death to heaven.

What does God say to us about life in heaven after we pass through the gate we call death?

1. He says that heaven is our true home.

> But our homeland is in heaven and it is from there
> that we are expecting a Savior, the Lord Jesus Christ.
>
> —PHILIPPIANS 3:20 NJB

We spend our lives this side of death, thinking this is all there is. Many of us enjoy most of it, but many others simply struggle to go on. The truth is, this part of life is only a preface to the real life, where we have been born to abide. When we reach the end of this phase of life and pass through the barbed gate of death, we are not entering a strange land—we are coming home.

2. He says that we will be transformed when we get there.

> Who, by the power that enables him to bring everything under his control, will transform our lowly bodies so that they will be like his glorious body.
>
> —PHILIPPIANS 3:21

Like many humans, I have never had the body I wanted and have fought to make it into what I imagined it could be. Even more so, as disease or age transforms my body into a more difficult cage, I will one day long to be released from weakness, pain, immobility, and insufficient strength. The truth is, I will be! One day our frail human bodies will be transformed into a body like that of Jesus himself, and we will keep that body forever.

3. He says our sadness will be gone.

> Never again will they hunger;
> never again will they thirst.
> The sun will not beat upon them,
> nor any scorching heat.
> For the Lamb at the center of the throne will be their shepherd;
> he will lead them to springs of living water.
> And God will wipe away every tear from their eyes.
>
> —REVELATION 7:16–17

For those of us who have lived long enough to know sadness in our lives, the thought of a life without tears seems like a dream. But the one who loves us enough to die for us would not promise us this dream and fail to fulfill it someday. His love is not an impotent love. He, himself, has torn down the gates to hell from where comes all of our sadness and has destroyed the pipeline that carries that sadness into our lives. His love is coupled with power. He will deliver what he has promised, and someday life will be filled only with happiness.

4. He says the joy of heaven will be God himself.

> Then I saw a new heaven and a new earth. . . . And I heard a loud voice from the throne saying, "Now the

> dwelling of God is with men, and he will live with them. They will be his people, and God himself will be with them and be their God."
>
> —REVELATION 21:1, 3

We have lived our lives at varying distances from our God. Sometimes it seems we are close to God; other times he seems far away. Perhaps now is one of those times when God seems far away. Try to think back to those times when you can remember his closeness, feel the sensation of his touch, see the evidence of his majesty, and feel the arms of his love. When we look back on those times, we realize that those were the times when life was its fullest—when it was really worth living in spite of circumstances about us. These moments of closeness to God come and go throughout our life on this side of death. Our moments of closeness to God here on earth are a mere shadow of what is to come. Such moments when we really know God will be continuous in heaven because that's what heaven is all about.

5. He says he will come himself to take us home.

> For the Lord himself will come down from heaven, with a loud command, with the voice of the archangel and with the trumpet call of God, and the dead in Christ will rise first. After that, we who are still alive and are left will be caught up together with them in the clouds to meet the Lord in the air. And so we will be with the Lord forever.
>
> —1 THESSALONIANS 4:16–17

Heaven sounds wonderful. But sometimes the thought of the journey we will take to get there is frightening. God promises we do not have to walk that journey alone. As we first turn the knob on the door marked "Death," Jesus himself will come down from heaven and walk us home. We need not fear the dark, for the Light of the World will show us the way. We need not fear the cliffs to nothingness, for the Good Shepherd will guide us safely along the path. The journey itself will be one of the sweetest things in life as we walk hand-in-hand with our Savior.

Not only that, but there is another key word in this passage from Paul to the Thessalonians. The word is *together*. Paul is saying that not only will we be walking home with our Savior but those we love, who love Jesus as well, will be walking with us. If our greatest dread of death is separation from those we love, we can throw that dread away. Death at first separates temporarily, like going off to work separates one from one's family, but death in Christ eventually unites forever.

A man I loved, who loved the Lord, was dying of cancer. He was unconscious and breathing irregularly. I informed his family that it would be but a few hours before he died. His daughter became overcome with uncontrollable grief and tears. The next day I entered the room and the patient was awake. He told me that the day before he had awakened to the sobbing of his daughter and had told her, "I was in heaven just now with Papa. It was wonderful. But I heard you crying, and I came back to comfort you. Now straighten up. I can't come back again. I love you." He died the next day with his family at peace. If heaven was where he could be with his Papa, someday his own children would again be with their father; and that day he would never have to leave them again. We, too, will be united again with those we love if they, too, love our Lord.

On my long, hot, painful run, it was the dream of the pool that kept me going. But the actual experience of those cool waters was a far greater joy than the dream. As you walk through a difficult life, the dream of heaven may sometimes be all that keeps you going. You can be confident that heaven is real, and someday the reality will be far greater than your dream.

When Cardinal Joseph Bernardin, the spiritual leader of Chicago's 2.3 million Catholics, discovered that his pancreatic cancer was not curable, he spoke publicly about facing death. He was quoted in our local paper, in an article by the Associated Press, saying, "I can say with all sincerity that I am at peace." He had been spending much of his time since his original cancer surgery counseling cancer patients "to place themselves entirely in the hands of the Lord." When his own cancer recurred, he said he would now take his own advice. Cardinal Bernardin knew that heaven was his home and that the hands of God were there to receive him and hold him. "We can look at death in two ways, as an enemy or as a friend," he said. "As a person of faith, I see death as a friend."

In the movie *Apollo 13,* Ed Harris was nominated for best supporting actor for his role as Gene Kranz, the man in charge of Houston Control. I believe he won that nomination for one critical scene. With the space capsule reentering the earth's atmosphere, the heat shields were damaged and battery power was down; there was little chance the astronauts would survive and reach earth alive. One officer at the Houston Center declared, "This is going to be the worst disaster that NASA has ever experienced," to which Kranz answered with determination in his jaw and a hint of defiance in his tone, "With all due respect, sir, I believe this is going to be our finest hour."[1]

So shall it be with death. Though the world tells us that death will be our greatest disaster, my patients and God's promise declare instead that death will become our finest hour.

IN THE MEANTIME

We started with the doctor's bad news, and we ended with life in heaven. That's the truth of our lives as Christians. But now the book is finished. It is time for you to get out there and live for as long a time as you have left on this earth. Is there some little thing you can carry in your hand as you live each day, each hour between the bad news and heaven, that you can look at quickly and know you are walking down the path he wants you to travel? Is there a map you can turn to that will keep you on God's road as you continue the race?

Sometimes we approach life too much like the way a boy named Jay used to approach Little League baseball. Coach Carson said he had never seen such talent in a ten-year-old boy. Jay could throw, hit, run, catch, and field—a natural. And yet, with all his ability, Jay always seemed to be out of position with his mind elsewhere.

I remember one day when his turn to catch fly balls came around. There he was, staring into space in the outfield. Coach Carson dropped his bat and walked out to confront the sky-gazer, who had not responded to his shouting.

"What are you doing out here, Jay, looking for geese?"

"No, Coach, I'm thinking about playing for the Padres. I'm going to be their starting shortstop someday," answered Jay with an excited grin across his face.

His coach couldn't help but smile at the young fellow's excitement, but he knew there was a problem. "Jay, if you want to be great, it's important to dream about it, but it's also important what you do *in the meantime.* Now turn around, pay attention, and catch these balls I'm hitting at you."

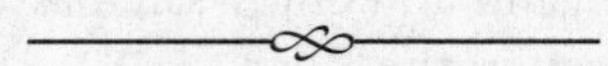

In the meantime probably is the most important place in life. Think about it. We spend most of our lives as goal-oriented people looking ahead to the next goal. When we reach that goal, we focus on the one after that, and the time between the goals is lost in a blur of expectation or preparation. In reality, life between the goals is where we truly live. Someone put it this way, "Life is what happens when you are waiting for the important." The fullness of life resides in the meantime.

When you hear the doctor's bad news, you have a choice. You can accept your tragic circumstance as the only important event left in life and waste your time focusing on it until heaven comes, or you can live life to its fullest in the meantime. I recently sat next to a man who had cancer in his liver and told him that no further treatment was available for his condition. He was in pretty good physical shape and could probably enjoy a decent quality of life for six months to one year. He looked at me and said, "You mean, Doc, that there is nothing else to do; I'm just waiting to die?" I told him there was no further worthwhile treatment but that he could choose whether he would just wait to die or live his life to the fullest in his remaining months. It's the same with you. Whatever the doctor's bad news, you can still choose to take the life God has given you and live it with passion and with purpose, completing what he has sent you here to do.

You can choose to live with passion and purpose, completing what God has sent you here to do.

What is it that God would have you do with the rest of your life after you have heard the doctor's bad news? It will all be fixed again in heaven someday, but what does God want you to do with yourself in the meantime?

God wants those of you who are broken in your health to live in the meantime the same way he wants everyone to live the rest of the time. He best summarizes his desire for our lives in one of David's songs:

> Trust in the Lord and do good;
> dwell in the land and enjoy safe pasture.
> Delight yourself in the Lord
> and he will give you the desires of your heart.
>
> —PSALM 37:3–4

This is the bottom line for life in this world. As all of us consider a life ahead that may be shorter than we had hoped and filled with more challenges than we desire, it is critical that we get back to the bottom line and use the rest of our life in the way it was intended.

Bad news awaits all of us—some sooner, some later. Regardless of the length of our remaining days or the physical difficulties within them, the Lord longs for us to live abundantly while we are on this side of heaven. He longs to give us the desires of our hearts. Let us trust him and do good. And even in the face of broken dreams or impending death, let us fall in love with God and live fully for him in the meantime.

> Soar we now where Christ has led,
> Following our exalted Head.
> Made like Him, like Him we rise,
> Ours the cross, the grave, the skies.[2]

Chapter Two—Choose God's Place in Your Crisis

1. Dale Matthews and Connie Clark, *Faith Factor: Proof of the Healing Power of Prayer* (New York: Penguin Putnam, 1998).
2. Ernest Becker, *The Denial of Death* (New York: Free Press Paperbacks, 1973), 26.
3. Michael Behe, *Darwin's Black Box* (New York: Touchstone, 1996), 74–97.
4. James Collier and Janie Buck, "Ruthless Trust," *Today's Christian Doctor* 30, no. 1 (spring 1999): 67.
5. Robert Ellsberg, *All Saints* (New York: Crossword, 1997), 131.

Chapter Three—Choose the Best Science

1. Donal O'Mathuna and Walt Larimore, *Alternative Medicine: The Christian Handbook* (Grand Rapids, Mich.: Zondervan, 2001).

Chapter Four—Choose Reality

1. Ellsberg, *All Saints,* 20.
2. *The Santa Clause* (Hollywood: Walt Disney Pictures, 1994).
3. Corrie ten Boom, *The Hiding Place* (Minneapolis: World Wide, 1971), 51.

Chapter Five—Choose to Help Shape Your Future

1. Jimmie C. Holland, et al., "Dealing with Loss, Death, and Grief in Clinical Practice: Spiritual Meaning in Oncology," *American Society of Clinical Oncology Educational Book* (Alexandria, Va.: ASCO, 2002), 198–205.

Chapter Six—Run to the God You Can Trust

1. David Waters, "Olympic Torch Flame Will Glow with Her Own Fiery Determination," *Commercial Appeal, (*25 November 2001), p. B1.
2. Source unknown.
3. Dietrich Bonhoeffer, *The Cost of Discipleship* (New York: Collier, Macmillan, 1963).
4. Phillip LeTard, *The Alaska Trip,* unpublished diary.

Chapter Eight—Choose to Face the Tough Questions

1. Ellsberg, *All Saints,* 12–13.
2. L. B. Cowman, *Streams in the Desert* (Grand Rapids, Mich.: Zondervan, 1977), 72.
3. Joni Eareckson Tada, "Medical Issues," Christian Doctor's Digest tape recording (Bristol, Tenn.: Christian Medical and Dental Society, December 1997).
4. Ibid.

Chapter Nine—Choose to Keep Praying

1. W. Somerset Maugham, *Of Human Bondage* (New York: Penguin, 1963), 53–55.
2. Pat Alger, Larry Bastian, and Garth Brooks, "Unanswered Prayers," *Garth Brooks: No Fences* (Nashville: Capital Records, 2000).
3. Harry Emerson Fosdick, *The Meaning of Prayer* (Nashville: Abingdon, 1981), 104.
4. Rex Warner, trans., *The Confessions of St. Augustine* (New York: Penguin, 1963), 101.

Chapter Ten—Choose Real Value

1. Don McLean, "Vincent," *The Best of Don McLean* (EMI, 1987).
2. Omar Khayyam, *Rubaiyat of Omar Khayyam* (Tehran: Padideh, n.d.).
3. William Barclay, *The Gospel of Matthew,* rev. ed., vol. 11 (Philadelphia: Westminster Press, 1975), 91.

Chapter Eleven—Choose to Pursue Joy

1. Dennis Linde, Bob Morrison, "The Love She Found in Me," *Gary Morris Hits* (Warner Brothers, 1983).
2. Kevin Robbins, "Classmates, Family Miss 'Shining Star,'" *Commercial Appeal (*17 February 1996), n.p.
3. William Barclay, *The Letters to the Philippians, Colossians, and Thessalonians* (Philadelphia: Westminster Press, 1975), 207.
4. Kevin Robbins, "In the End, Somthing Beautiful," *Commercial Appeal (*26 November 1995), pp. E1–2.

Chapter Thirteen—Choose to Pursue Peace

1. Kevin Robbins, "In the End, Something Beautiful," *Commercial Appeal (*26 November 1995), pp. E1–2.
2. Murray Alexander, a letter to his family, used with permission.

Chapter Fifteen—Choose Mission

1. Dietrich Bonhoeffer, *Letters and Papers from Prison* (New York: Macmillan, 1953), 197.

Chapter Eighteen—Anticipate Your Future

1. *Apollo 13* (Universal City, Calif.: Universal City Studios, 1995).
2. Charles Wesley, "Christ the Lord Is Risen Today."

Christian Medical Association
Resources

Medically reliable ... biblically sound. That's the rock-solid promise of this series offered by Zondervan in partnership with the Christian Medical Association. Each book in this series is not only written by fully credentialed, experienced doctors but is also fully reviewed by an objective board of qualified doctors to ensure its reliability. Because when your health is at stake, you can't settle for anything less than the whole and accurate truth.

Integrating your faith and health can improve your physical well-being and even extend your life, as you gain insights into the interconnection of health and faith-a relationship largely overlooked by secular science. Benefit from the cutting-edge knowledge of respected medical experts as they help you make health care decisions consistent with your beliefs. Their sound biblical analysis of emerging treatments and technologies equips you to protect yourself from seemingly harmless-yet spiritually, ethically, or medically unsound-options and then to make the healthiest choices possible.

Through this series, you can draw from both the knowledge of science and the wisdom of God's Word in addressing your medical ethics decisions and in meeting your health care needs.

Founded in 1931, the Christian Medical Association helps thousands of doctors minister to their patients by imitating the Great Physician, Jesus Christ. Christian Medical Association members provide a Christian voice on medical ethics to policy makers and the media, minister to needy patients on medical missions around the world, evangelize and disciple students on more than 90 percent of the nation's medical school campuses, and provide educational and inspirational resources to the church.

To learn more about Christian Medical Association ministries and resources on health care and ethical issues, browse the website (www.christianmedicalassociation.org) or call toll-free at 888-231-2637.

"Dear friend, I pray that you may enjoy good health and that all may go well with you, even as your soul is getting along well."

(3 John 2 NIV)

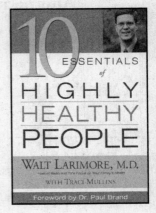

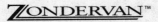

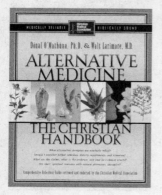

Jesus, M.D.

A Doctor Examines the Great Physician

David Stevens, M.D.,
with Gregg Lewis

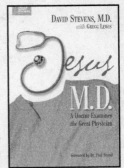

Jesus—the ultimate doctor. His touch extended grace to the sick and sinful of ancient Palestine and left a miracle in its wake. And his ministry hasn't ceased. Today, he looks for willing hearts and hands through which he can heal a needy world.

Dr. David Stevens knows. His eleven years at Tenwek Hospital in Kenya have shown him more than the drama and sacrifice of missionary medicine. In *Jesus, M.D.* Dr. Stevens shares the insights he has gained into the character, power, and purposes of the Great Physician and what it means for *you* to follow in his footsteps.

This is more than a book of dramatic, true-life stories. It is an inspiring and challenging invitation to partner with Jesus in his "practice," accompanying him on his rounds to people whose lives he wants to make whole. Discover how to participate with him in bringing his healing touch to your corner of the world. You don't need a medical education—just determination to trust God as your "attending physician," your mentor, and your source of guidance, discipline, and encouragement.

Dr. Stevens takes you inside stories from the Bible to obtain challenging perspectives and life-changing truths. You'll also get an inside look at life-or-death surgeries; the tense, powerful relationship between resident and attending physicians; the overcrowded patient quarters of a missionary hospital; what it's like to improvise an emergency facial reconstruction; and much more. Best of all, you'll gain surprising insights from the life and methods of Jesus, the ultimate doctor, in his ministry to desperately needy people two thousand years ago . . . and today.

Electrifying, moving, and thought-provoking, *Jesus, M.D.* will help you see your relationship with God and your world in a brand-new light. Your life is filled with incredible possibilities waiting to unfold one by one as you walk in the presence and provision of Dr. Jesus.

Some books address the health of our bodies. Others nurture the mind. A few of them have a story to tell. Still others touch the soul. This one brings all of these strengths with profound and practical wisdom.

Ravi Zacharias
President, Ravi Zacharias International Ministries

Hardcover: 0-310-23433-6

Pick up a copy at your favorite bookstore today!